HEALING FROM THE INSIDE OUT

Overcome Chronic Disease and Radically Change Your Life

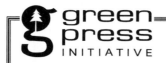
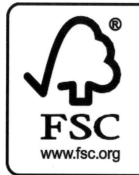

HEALING FROM THE INSIDE OUT

Overcome Chronic Disease and Radically Change Your Life

NAUMAN NAEEM MD

 FINDHORN PRESS

Published in 2017 by Findhorn Press, Scotland

ISBN 978-1-84409-736-4

Edited by Nicky Leach
Cover photo (butterfly) by Greg Hurley
Cover design by Richard Crookes
Interior design by Damian Keenan
Printed and bound in the USA

DISCLAIMER

The information in this book (in print and electronic media)
is given in good faith and is neither intended to diagnose any
physical or mental condition nor to serve as a substitute for
informed medical advice or care.
Please contact your health professional for medical advice and
treatment. Neither author nor publisher can be held liable by
any person for any loss or damage whatsoever which may arise
from the use of this book or any of the information therein.

Published by
Findhorn Press
117-121 High Street,
Forres IV36 1AB,
Scotland, UK

t +44 (0)1309 690582
f +44 (0)131 777 2711
e info@findhornpress.com
www.findhornpress.com

Contents

FOREWORD

by Bernie Siegel, MD
Author of *Love, Medicine, and Miracles*

It was a pleasure for me to read Dr. Naeem's book, because I agree with him. Decades ago, I tried to get our message out to patients and medical professionals and was told I was giving false hope and blaming my patients by asking them what was going on in their life. What they were referring to is that I did not treat patients as a statistic and tell them when they would die. I let them know their potential. People do win the lottery and survive so-called incurable illnesses.

I also inquired into people's lives to see if they were vulnerable to a disease due to stressful events and changes in their lives. I know from personal experience that you can't separate your life and emotions from your health. Monday mornings are an example of that.

Our emotions create our body chemistry: just as laughter can improve survival, hopelessness and depression can reduce our chances of staying healthy and surviving. Blood tests done on actors revealed that reading a comedy script enhanced their immune function and lowered stress hormone levels, while acting out a tragedy had the opposite effect. And in a study of cancer patients, those who laughed for no apparent reason several times a day had a better survival rate than the control group who did not laugh for no reason.

Doctors are trained to treat the resulting diagnosis and not the cause. Drug advertisements tell you what pill to take for your diagnosis and never mention your life's circumstances and healing them. We need to treat each patient's experience and not just prescribe but help them heal their lives. Mother Teresa told a group who invited her that she would not attend an anti-war rally, "but if you ever have a peace rally, call me." We need to help patients do what this book is about; to heal their lives, minds, and bodies, because people are a unit and not a mechanical object.

When we wage a war against cancer and other diseases, we empower the enemy. Utilizing love and faith can heal lives and bodies. I know people who accepted their mortality and left their troubles to God or went to beautiful places to enjoy their last few months of life and then didn't die. Two of their quotes are: "It was so beautiful here I forgot to die" and "I didn't die, and now I'm so busy I'm killing myself. Help. Where do I go from here?"

Songwriters, poets, and novelists view the world and write about it from their experience. W.H. Auden, in his poem "Miss Gee," has a doctor say to his wife, over dinner, after examining a lonely woman that day and discovering cancer:

> *Cancer's a funny thing...*
> *Childless women get it.*
> *And men when they retire;*
> *It's as if there had to be some outlet*
> *for their foiled creative fire.*

A doctor yelled at me after I said this during a lecture, "Just because it rhymes doesn't make it true." But it is true, and we know this today. Elida Evans, a Jungian therapist in the 1930s, wrote in her book, "Cancer is growth gone wrong. A message to take a new road in your life."

This is not about guilt, blame, and shame but about becoming a responsible participant in your health and life and not just a submissive sufferer or so-called "good patient."

For many people, this is a problem due to the guilt related to religions and parenting. When you grow up with the opposite of love—indifference, rejection, and abuse—you're a prime candidate for serious illness. A study of Harvard students showed that those who didn't feel loved by their parents had a 98 percent serious illness rate by middle age, and those who felt loved had only a 24 percent serious illness rate.

Religions and clergy can add to the problem patients have, when they believe and say that God may give people cancer to bring them back to the church when they lose contact with their religion. An example is the message from Pope Leo XI to Catholics in 1823. He said that God decides who gets smallpox, so if you vaccinate yourself you won't go to Heaven since you are no longer a child of God. Things have changed, but that guilt-laden thinking can still remain, and I hear it from modern day clergy, too.

Maimonides, a thousand years ago, said two things that make the truth clear. One, that disease is a loss of health, and we are all here to do as the Bible tells us and help our neighbor find what he has lost. Second, that if people took as good care of themselves as they do of their animals they would suffer fewer illnesses.

How true those statements still are today. We all need to love ourselves, our lives, and our bodies and take as good care of ourselves as we do of our beloved pets. I know of one couple who, when their cats developed lung cancer and breathing problems, wrote a column in *Cat Fancy* magazine that finishes with: "Doug and I now smoke in the yard. We are not killing our cats anymore. We hope you're not killing yours."

He who seeks to save his life will lose it, while he who is willing to lose his life will save it. When you become submissive and give up your desires and happiness to please others you lose your life, and when you wake up to that fact and heal and reclaim your life, amazing things can happen emotionally and physically. The submissive twin sister who tries to make her parents happy while denying her needs is far more likely to develop breast cancer than her independent little devil of a sister who lets her heart make up her mind.

Years ago, when I started a cancer support group called EcaP (Exceptional Cancer Patients), they became my teachers. The label "exceptional" came from the fact that after sending one hundred letters to my patients offering them a support group and a longer better life, only twelve women showed up.

Women do have better survival rates than men with the same cancers, and married men do better than single men due to their relationships. But the majority of men with cancer are more likely to die when they can't work anymore. Then their life loses all meaning because they are living a role not an authentic life, and when they can't work their life loses its meaning. I have had men in my office, sitting with their wife and children say, "There's no point in living, I can't work anymore." I point out their family sitting next to them as a reason. One man committed suicide after his doctor said, "You can't work, sail your boat, or play tennis anymore." I also learned a great deal from Elisabeth Kubler-Ross and started using my patients' dreams and drawings to help them understand what their consciousness was trying to tell them.

I thought I was learning about and uncovering amazing things and so wrote articles and sent them to medical journals to enlighten everyone. The medical journals sent them back with a note saying they were interesting "but not appropriate for our journal." So I sent them to psychiatry and psychology journals, and again they were returned, but this time the note said that they were appropriate but not interesting.

Medicine departmentalizes people as if they are mechanical objects, when they are not. Mind and body are a unit. Psychiatrists are more aware of this because they see the physical benefits of their work. When I wrote my first book, I sent a copy to psychiatrist Dr. Karl Menninger to read. He wrote me a letter back, saying he was about to write a book about ten hopeless cases who were alive and well today, "but I am not going to write it because you just did."

Psychiatrists formulate terms like Immune Competent Personality. They know the power of the mind and what I have labeled "deceiving people into health." You can call it a placebo or hypnotic effect, but the mind can do amazing things with the body. I also see people who, due to medical errors, have not received their cancer treatments, but their doctors did not realize it until routine inspections were done and uncovered the mistake because their patients all acted as if they were being treated due to their beliefs.

After drawing pictures for Kubler-Ross, I began to ask my patients to draw pictures for me and questioned them about their dreams. These are not things that are a part of a medical education, although they are established sources of information about the body, the disease, and the treatment.

I have been able to diagnose people's illnesses from their drawings alone and have written books about this, because I am familiar with anatomy while an art therapist is not and can miss the information in the drawings. Asking a patient to draw themselves, their disease, their treatment, and their immune system eliminating their illness is a useful tool in helping patients make the right choices about their health. For example, drawing the devil giving you poison is not a good sign for a patient undergoing chemotherapy.

Our intuitive wisdom and intellect need to communicate with each other and help us to make the right decisions for ourselves. Doctors need to be taught about a patient's potential and help them to achieve it. I have never met a medical student who, while in medical school, was told that Carl Jung diagnosed a brain tumor from a patient's dream. We need to share the information and open the minds of healthcare providers and their patients.

The word "potential" means a lot to me because I try to teach people about survivor behavior. When I began to meet people at my lectures whom I thought had died, I always asked them how come they didn't die, and they all had stories to tell about changes they made in their lives. We need to spread the word and let people know that they are not statistics. Doctors can kill or cure with their words. I learned that wordswordswords can become swordswordswords and can kill or cure the patient.

When a patient recovers from a so-called "incurable disease," it is not a spontaneous remission; it is a case of self-induced healing. It is always related to their rebirthing themselves and their lives and finding a rhythm and harmony in their life they never experienced before. When you love your life and body, amazing things happen. Russian author Alexander Solzhenitsyn discusses this in his novel *Cancer Ward*, which introduced me to the term "self-induced healing," a term you never hear a doctor use. In this book, the symbol of the healing is a rainbow-colored butterfly.

We need to stop training doctors to treat the result and not the cause. Nauman Naeem's book will help you to personally accomplish that. We need to understand not just the diagnosis but what the patients are experiencing and help them to heal their lives and bodies.

The meaning of the word "patient" is derived from a submissive sufferer. So if you are a good hospitalized patient, you are more likely to die due to medical errors because people don't know you. They see you as a diagnosis or room number and not a person. I want all of you who read this book to be empowered and instead of being good patients become "respants" (responsible participants).

As physicians, we must awaken to the fact that our job is to do more than just treat a disease. We need to become a resource and life coach for our patients and see them in a sense as our children who need guidance, love, hope, and an education about being a survivor. I have learned that there is no false hope. Hope is real; it is not about statistics but about people being reborn and giving their body a live message, which it responds to, knowing that life is a gift and not a diagnosis.

So read on, and let Naeem's book coach and redirect you onto a life healing path. There is nothing to fear. This is not about being a failure if everything doesn't work out or a miracle doesn't happen, or being afraid to draw a picture because you are not an artist, or not having time to read a book. This is about being open to coaching, changing your life, and healing from the inside out. Our creator has given us the potential, so step up and activate your inner resources.

Introduction

This book is the culmination of several threads that have interwoven and defined my life from the time I was a child.

I was born in London, England, and lived there for a short time before my parents immigrated to Toronto, Canada. I remember having a voracious appetite for knowledge and soaking up everything I could learn from school, books, newspapers, my elders, and many other sources. I felt it was my duty and privilege to gain as much knowledge as I could about many spheres of life.

Another defining thread in my early childhood was my thirst for adventure and the feeling that without an element of risk, life becomes mundane and routine.

This played out in my childhood in various ways. I would bike farther from my neighborhood than I did the week before. I would trace the creek close to my house along its tributary until it flowed into the larger river. I would follow train tracks for miles and I would do many other things that I hoped my parents would never find out about. Then, as I reached adolescence, my sense of adventure manifested in other ways, as I dabbled in various pursuits, from hiking, camping, and skiing to whitewater rafting, windsurfing, and rock climbing.

I grew up in a predominantly white blue collar neighborhood and city, east of Toronto, and was the only south Asian kid in both elementary and high school. I often felt myself caught between the worlds of my Muslim south Asian culture and Western culture. This was a struggle that played out both at home and in school, as I wanted to fit in with my peers while maintaining my cultural identity.

I faced a lot of racial discrimination but was able to maintain a few close friendships throughout high school. In spite of this, I never lost the feeling that I was an outsider amongst my peers, even when I succumbed to peer pressure in order to be a part of the in crowd. I was caught between two worlds, and for most of my adolescence, was not able to reconcile them, so I had to choose one or the other most of the time. This created an inner conflict that has become a defining feature of my life's journey as it has unfolded over time.

As I transitioned from high school to university, I got busier with my studies and trying to forge a career path and gradually lost my sense of adventure. Seeking knowledge also began to lose its luster, as learning became more about getting the best grades to position myself competitively to enter the best graduate or professional schools.

Medicine piqued my interest during these years because it integrated science, service to humanity, and working with people, and although I applied to medical school, getting accepted was very competitive, and I failed to get into a Canadian medical school, two years in a row. Having completed my undergraduate studies, now I was more lost than ever.

I did odd jobs for a year after graduating before a new opportunity arose to attend an international medical school. That feeling of adventure and desire for knowledge was rekindled, as I was off to a foreign country to study medicine, experience a different culture, and learn a new language.

As exciting as this was, it was accompanied by a certain degree of uncertainty, because I would likely not be able to return to Canada to do postgraduate residency training, due to strict rules and regulations preventing international medical graduates from coming back to Canada. In order to do the same in the United States, I would have to pass a set of three medical licensing exams and secure a special visa permit which, at that time, was not easy to obtain.

This uncertainty, which caused so much fear and dread at that time, would eventually turn out to be a source of inspiration and a guiding force in my life, as you will learn later in this book. Nevertheless, I managed to overcome these obstacles, and got accepted into an internal medicine residency position in Cleveland, Ohio, in the United States. By this time, I was married, and as I continued my medical training in my residency program, I began to apply the knowledge I had gained in medical school to real-life clinical situations.

I seemed to be thriving on the outside, as I was well on my way to establishing a successful medical career, but there was something missing and, at that time, I had no idea what it was. I felt an emptiness. This motivated me to pursue a "spiritual search," and this became the third thread that came to define my life.

I delved deeply into books by such luminous spiritual authors as Wayne Dyer, Deepak Chopra, Neale Donald Walsch, and Eckhart Tolle, among others. My spiritual seeking continued as I entered my fellowship in Pulmonary and Critical Care medicine in Cleveland, and although I gained a lot from the books I read and the CDs I listened to, I still was not entirely sure what I was looking for.

I eventually finished my training and relocated to Northwest Ohio, where I entered into practice as a specialist in pulmonary and critical care. I cared for the sickest patients in the hospital, including those with respiratory failure, cardiac arrest, septic shock, massive heart attacks and strokes, kidney failure, gastrointestinal bleeding, advanced cancer, drug overdose, and many other life-threatening conditions. Some of these patients would not survive their acute illness and, in my career to date, I have witnessed more death than a seasoned war veteran. Witnessing so much death has greatly humbled me and given me a deep reverence for all that we hold sacred in our earthly life. However, it has also forced me to ask some deep and probing questions and to spend years trying to answer them.

Why do patients get so critically ill? Are they at fault? Is it due to their own neglect of their health? There are patients who do not follow their family physician's treatment regimens and recommendations, but why do patients end up living with chronic disease in the first place? Are we all destined to become chronically ill, barely managing symptoms with a host of pharmaceuticals, most of which cause side effects, and to eventually end up in the emergency department when the symptoms become unbearable and admitted to hospital?

As I struggled with trying to find answers to these questions, I began to look more closely at the patients I was caring for and started to recognize patterns. Upon further questioning patients and their families, I found that the vast majority of patients dealing with chronic disease and critical illness had personal stories behind their illness and showed unresolved issues from their past.

Now, this may not come as a surprise to most people, as the link between our thoughts and emotions and overall health has become well established.

What is surprising, though, is that the world's various healthcare systems have not embraced this notion and developed ways of addressing these issues as they pertain to health and chronic disease, especially since the cost of healthcare in the West has been rising exponentially in recent decades. I confirmed this for myself when I moved back to Ontario, Canada, to continue my pulmonary and critical care career, and noticed the same patterns there.

I was still on my "spiritual quest," but there too I began to question things. I was seeking the answers to life's most important questions by reading various books on healing, consciousness, and metaphysics and listening to numerous transformational and spiritual teleseminars, but what I was looking for still eluded me.

At the same time, I found myself wanting to rekindle that sense of adventure I had had as a child and became interested in self-reliance. During the last few years I lived in Ohio, I began fulfilling this interest by learning wilderness survival and primitive living skills from various mentors. This eventually led me down a path of deep nature connection, mainly through learning the ancient art of tracking.

Tracking is, in simple terms, scrutinizing your environment to come up with a story of what transpired in that environment, with the main application being animal tracking. This involves looking at the impressions that animals leave in various terrains and determining the species, its gait, how fast it was moving, and looking for other signs, such as browsing, scat, any prey remains from predation, and dens.

As I delved further into tracking, I became more deeply aware not only of the world around me but also my inner world emerging. My mentors confirmed this, noting that the growing awareness that comes from practicing the skill of tracking inevitably shines a bright light on the inner world of one's thoughts, emotions, and true essence—what some call "spirit" or "soul."

My own journey to self-awareness has not been a defined process with a distinct endpoint but has continued to grow and evolve. It has helped illuminate subconscious blocks, unresolved emotional pain, and limiting beliefs that I have held deep in my psyche. As I recognized the dual nature of my existence—that of a physical being on this earth and the deeper essence, being, presence, or consciousness that transcends my physical form—a whole new dimension of life that I scarcely knew existed has opened up.

This exploration of my inner realms nicely wove together the three threads in my life, as I realized the greatest knowledge is self-knowledge, the greater adventure is the journey to the core of one's being, and that one's spiritual search culminates in the discovery of one's true nature, which is that of pure consciousness. This was truly liberating as it instilled in me the sense of where real freedom lies, something that had eluded me since childhood, and shed new light on the nature of existence.

The path that led me to this inner tracking and deeper self-awareness was that of deep nature connection; however, the same can be achieved through many other means, including meditation, prayer, tai chi, yoga, long-distance running, creating artwork, playing music, singing, writing poetry, journaling and a whole host of other endeavors.

Through my inner tracking, I began to recognize patterns in my thoughts and emotions and how they would manifest in the physical realm.

For example, if I was worried about some task that I needed to accomplish in my daily routine, such as having a difficult conversation with a co-worker or peer, my worry would soon be validated. If, instead, I focused on only the most positive outcome that could arise from any task I need to complete, that would usually come to pass. Now, this is not a book about the power of positive thinking, but I just wanted to highlight how powerful our inner environment is in determining the nature of our outer experience.

As I continued to contemplate the relationship between our inner and outer reality, the knowledge of how we can truly heal suddenly became illuminated for me. This was not a sudden lightning bolt of insight; instead, it has been a gradual process, one that has unfolded over many years. I realized that the reason that people don't heal is because modern medicine's approach to treating chronic disease revolves around largely external means, namely pharmaceuticals and procedure-based therapies, including surgery.

This mirrors most people's approach to fulfillment in their lives: they think they can achieve satisfaction through accumulating more material things and more experiences, more entertainment, more travel, more socializing, more sexual gratification, and so forth. What they soon realize, though, is that the sole pursuit of external fulfillment leaves us emptier than we were when we started, just as the sole pursuit of external solutions to chronic illness leaves us with a well-managed chronic illness but not true healing.

The missing ingredient has always been establishing a balanced approach that includes both the inner and outer realms. Medications, procedure-based therapies, and surgeries are needed and often beneficial, but not to the exclusion of a focus on our inner life, which includes scrutiny of our thoughts, emotions, and an identification with our true nature.

What do I mean by our true nature? Many people believe that we are our physical bodies and buy into this illusion.

Why is this an illusion?

If we break down who we truly are at the physical level, we realize that we are made up of cells, which are made up of cellular organelles, which are made up of molecules, which are made up of atoms, which are made up of subatomic particles. And what are subatomic particles? They are just packets of energy vibrating at a certain frequency that emanate from our core essence or being.

So, if we break down who we are into our fundamental elements, we are just pure energy that can be transformed and transmuted, which means that anything is possible, including perfect health.

This may seem incredible to most people. But that is because we have spent most of our lives buying into the illusion of our false nature. We have become complacent in accepting outcomes in our lives without questioning their validity, especially when it comes to our health.

This book examines in a popular way how to bridge the gap between the inner and outer aspects of our health in order to achieve true healing. The ideas expressed are not a substitute for conventional medical care, and I do not recommend that anyone stop seeing their physicians or stop taking their medications. As noted, I am myself an allopathic physician and treat my patients with medications, if needed. A balanced approach is needed, however, in order to optimize our health and to heal at all levels.

At this point, I want to make a distinction between healing and cure. When I talk about healing in this book, I am not referring to cure. I am referring to integrating your being at all levels—physical, mental, emotional, vibrational, spiritual, and existential. This will create the optimal internal and external environment for your illness to be treated most effectively, with an improvement and, possibly, an elimination of your symptoms.

Before we go any farther, I must warn you that this book will challenge all your previous held beliefs and assumptions about health, healing, and chronic disease and force you to look deep within yourself to find the truth. On the other hand, it may awaken something deep within you that has lain dormant and obscured from the time of your birth.

This book is not so much about giving you new information, since I draw upon many other sources that have inspired me; however, I do introduce new ideas and concepts that I have not seen discussed elsewhere in the context of healing. My aim is to create a paradigm shift in your thinking about how to heal from chronic disease through opening your mind and heart to a more expansive and multidimensional way of seeing yourself and your world.

My intention in writing this book is to unveil and awaken you to your true nature. It is inevitable that the ideas expressed here will generate resistance, as they challenge the status quo; they may even be seen as threatening by mainstream medicine, which thrives on keeping patients chronically ill and dependent on the establishment.

Nevertheless, I feel that these ideas must be read, scrutinized, embodied, and shared with others for true healing to occur, both individually and globally. Fasten your seatbelts, because you are about to go on an incredible journey.

NOTE: At the end of each chapter, you will find Key Points, a summary of that chapter's main ideas, followed by Questions To Ask Your Clients. Although this book is for the general public, for those of you who are physicians, healthcare practitioners, health and wellness coaches, and healers, I have included these questions as diagnostic and therapeutic tools to use with clients or for self-reflection and to ignite your own healing process.

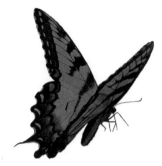

PART ONE

BACKGROUND TO THE HEALING PROCESS

CHAPTER 1

Your Illness Is a Gift

It may sound paradoxical to say that your illness is a gift, but there can be no deeper truth than this.

As an internal medicine, pulmonary, critical care, and palliative care physician, I have treated thousands of patients with issues as minor as a nagging cough to life-threatening issues, including actively dying patients, and there is a common thread that I find in most patients when I delve deeper: they have been living their lives on the outside, with little care or concern for the deeper aspects of their being.

Most individuals who examine their lives more closely will find this to be true. Illness, therefore, is a wake-up call to journey within. This is a step toward psychological and emotional healing that will ultimately help heal the physical illness.

When we are first born into this world, we are as pure as we will ever be, and our true nature shines forth onto the world. Anyone who has looked into the eyes of a newborn baby will know this to be true. There is no ego or false self; just the beauty of divine love in those eyes.

As the newborn grows up in its environment, it gets exposed to all sorts of stimuli, not all of which are perceived as positive. Maybe baby woke up one time in her crib and did not see her parents nearby. She may then have perceived that she was all alone, with nobody to care for her and began to cry. When this happened, maybe the parents did not respond to her cries right away, and there was a delay before she was picked up and consoled. A fear of abandonment was thereby imprinted in her mind for the first time.

As she enters childhood, then adolescence, followed by adulthood, this baby's childhood memory will offer an immediate frame of reference when she is faced with a similar situation. An example of this could be when a child is not picked up on time from a dance rehearsal, the same feelings of abandonment will resurface and cause distress and anxiety. Another example from adulthood could be when the child has a scheduled social engagement with a close friend or an acquaintance and, for some reason, that person does not show up. Again, the feelings of abandonment will come up, and the same emotions will surface.

Now, we are only talking about the simplest of emotionally distressing scenarios here. Imagine the emotional issues that are created in children who witness alcoholism at home; experience physical or sexual abuse or bullying; who are not able to make friends at school; who are made to feel inferior because of their ethnicity, their weight, their height, or a number of other physical characteristics; or who simply have one traumatic experience that forever colors their perception of the world in a negative way.

I cannot think of anyone who has not been negatively affected emotionally at some level by a stressful event that happened in their past. If you sit down and question people you know in depth, you will be able to tease out at least one such historical event in everyone. It does not have to be something as major as physical or sexual abuse; it could be as simple as the school scenario I mentioned above.

The problem is that the human mind catalogs every experience as a memory and creates a frame of reference that triggers similar emotions when we face even remotely similar scenarios at other times in our lives. Experiences that cause emotional trauma can be referred to as "wounds." Nobody who is born into this world is immune from wounds. We all experience them at some level or another.

It is not just children and adolescents who experience wounds. Think of all the challenges we face as adults—relationship issues, separation, divorce, job loss, geographic moves, death of a family member. And these are just the major issues. Countless minor issues permeate our daily life, too, including arguments at work, job stress, rush hour traffic, paying the bills, balancing the household budget, picking up the kids from school on time, planning dinner, and so forth.

These can all cause emotional stress which, if not navigated effectively, can result in minor wounds that add up to cause significant health challenges. In fact, many healthcare professionals have recognized stress as a major health challenge in modern times.

The main problem is that children are not usually taught how to manage the stresses of daily life. As we grow into adolescents and young adults, our responsibilities increase, along with the demands on our time, which results in an exponential increase in our stress level, and there is never any formal education on how to deal with stress.

We are left to our own devices to manage our stress, which eventually evolves into chronic anxiety. People utilize many methods to handle this nervous tension. Some may be healthy, such as meditation, yoga, exercise, going for contemplative walks, and reading; others not as healthy, such as smoking, using alcohol and other illicit substances, overeating, and numerous other unhealthy means.

The problem is that these unhealthy means of handling stress may relieve the issues briefly, but they never provide any permanent solutions. This leads to an increase in the frequency of the negative habit, which, in addition to the original stress, leads to chronic health issues. Unless these issues are dealt with at the core, even positive ways of alleviating stress only serve to temporarily sugarcoat our underlying nervous tension and anxieties.

So why is your illness a gift?

Your illness is a gift because it points to disruption at the core of your being, a deeper level than the outer physical symptoms manifested by the illness. If you have the insight and courage to take this journey, your illness can force you to go down the rabbit hole and uncover all the hidden recesses of your inner world and illuminate the true cause of your disease. The problem is that most people do not realize this and, if they do, do not have the tools or the courage to take this journey within.

KEY POINTS

- All illnesses are symptoms of core issues that we need to resolve.
- Everyone suffers from these core issues at some level.

CHAPTER 2

THE HEART OF THE MATTER

The treatment of illness has evolved mainly in the realm of the physical. With the advent of modern medicine, a recent phenomenon, we have developed the ability to treat conditions that, in the past, would have killed most people.

Examples include antibiotics for infections, dialysis for kidney failure, angioplasty and coronary artery bypass grafting for heart attacks, mechanical ventilation for respiratory failure, organ transplant for the failure of many organs, not to mention the countless pharmaceuticals that are available for the treatment of almost any medical condition out there.

Modern treatments have revolutionized the practice of medicine, allowing patients to live longer with chronic disease. But these advances bring with them a burden of suffering for everyone afflicted with chronic illness, right from the early stages of the disease.

This burden includes:

Living with ongoing symptoms that often cause physical and emotional pain and stress, because the disease is only being managed, not eliminated.

Having to take expensive daily medications, with the associated cost to the individual (and to society, if they are paid for by employer or government benefits).

Wasted time from having to regularly visit your family physician and specialists to help manage your chronic disease, and the loss of income from having to take time off work for these visits.

The risk of your condition worsening, requiring you to go to the emergency room and potentially be admitted to the hospital for acute treatments. This means further costs for the individual, not only from the hospitalization but also from lost time at work.

If you are hospitalized, the loss of income for family members and friends who have to take time off work to regularly visit you.

The added stress and uncertainty of being hospitalized, which only compounds the original condition that led to the hospitalization.

The social cost of hospitalization, if your healthcare coverage is through a government program such as Medicare or Medicaid in the United States. If you have private healthcare insurance, hospitalization results in rising premiums for everyone, adding to the overall cost of delivering healthcare.

The added costs of recovering from a hospitalization, which often include physical rehabilitation programs, transfer to chronic care facilities, and post-hospitalization home-care services.

The added burden of disability from chronic diseases such as diabetes, heart disease, and cancer.

The grief and suffering caused to the loved ones of individuals who die from chronic diseases, which account for 7 out of 10 deaths in the United States alone.[1]

These are just a few of the burdens that chronic disease places on individuals who suffer from them and on society at large. If we look strictly at the annual financial costs of chronic disease in the United States alone, the numbers are staggering; heart disease and stroke cost $432 billion, diabetes costs $174 billion, lung disease costs $154 billion, and Alzheimer's Disease costs $148 billion.[2,3,4,5] These social, emotional, and financial costs are a direct result of our healthcare culture, which emphasizes management of chronic disease and not dealing with the root causes of illness.

Where do these root causes of illness lie? Is it in our genetics, our eating habits, our lack of exercise, smoking, drinking tainted tap water, breathing polluted air, or the numerous other environmental toxins that we are continuously exposed to?

Certainly all of these factors contribute to ill health; however, they don't get to the heart of the matter. Addressing these external issues can help to alleviate the symptoms of chronic illness and improve one's health, but unless the core issues at the heart of all chronic diseases are addressed, complete healing will not occur.

At core, all chronic diseases are rooted in loss of identity. What do I mean by loss of identity?

As already mentioned, we come into this world as pure love and light, born from the realm of the absolute into the realm of the relative. This means that we are born into a world in which we can experience the full spectrum of human experiences, ranging from the pit of despair and hopelessness to the heights of elation and ecstasy.

As we navigate the maze of human life, we are bound to experience seemingly negative experiences because this is a part of everyone's journey in physical form. The unfortunate thing is that as these negative experiences accumulate over time, they begin to obscure our original nature of pure love and light. We start to identify with these experiences and take them on as an identity.

This is the origin of subconscious blocks and limiting beliefs. Our true nature infuses and animates all aspects of our being, including our emotions, our minds, and bodies, but as it becomes obscured, every aspect of our being becomes adversely affected. This is what causes diseases of the emotions, such as depression; diseases of the mind, such as anxiety; and diseases of the body—all of which are too familiar to us all.

An example of how negative experiences can affect our physiology is takotsubo cardiomyopathy, a heart condition that has been acknowledged by cardiologists worldwide. This is a severe dysfunction of the main large chamber of the heart, the left ventricle. Its cause is unknown but has been attributed to a significant emotional stressor in the patient's life.

So why do we go through life accumulating layer upon layer of emotional traumas, which lead to subconscious blocks and limiting beliefs, followed by emotional, psychological, and physical symptoms, chronic disease, ongoing suffering and, eventually, a miserable death? If we look at the ways in which society trains and manipulates the masses and leads most of us down a path of sorrow, struggle, and hopelessness, the reasons become clear.

Traditional education systems, which is what most of us have been exposed to, focus on rote learning and regurgitating facts; they leave out the skills that really matter and that can lead to true prosperity and happiness—conveying true unconditional love and compassion, achieving inner peace, experiencing pure awareness, radiating joy, and expressing gratitude. These and similar life skills should be taught early in life at all of our educational institutions, so that we never lose sight of our true nature.

Now, don't get me wrong. Reading, writing, math, science, history, geography, social sciences, art, music, and physical education are all important subjects for our children to learn, but not at the expense of the life skills I have mentioned above.

If we can teach kids to master life skills like expressing unconditional love and maneuvering through adversity with inner calm, they will be happier, healthier, enthusiastic, inspired, and able to learn their other school subjects effortlessly and with great joy. This is because their true nature will always shine through, no matter what situation they face and what obstacles are placed before them in their life situation.

These life skills have not yet been subjected to rigorous research due to the inherent difficulty in objectively measuring unconditional love, inner peace, sincere gratitude, and true joy; however, when we take time to consider them, the benefits seem intuitive. Who is a better learner—someone who has learnt self-calming skills and the ability to express unconditional love and joy or someone who is depressed, miserable, and bitter?

Even though our educational institutions do not reinforce these values, one would hope that our children are being taught these values at home. Unfortunately, this is not true in the majority of cases. Parents are often working longer hours in stressful workplaces in order to maintain a standard of living whose cost has increased over the last several decades. This means that they are not always there to guide their children in difficult times nor to teach them the values they need in order to lead healthy, balanced, and successful lives.

Furthermore, parents themselves lose sight of their own true nature as they identify with their life experiences, with the result that they find themselves incapable of guiding their children through the complexities of life in the physical plane.

This was once a sacred role in indigenous cultures. The elders of the tribe would raise young children and guide them through the different stages of their growth and development, from infancy through young adulthood, using nature as the backdrop in which to nurture this growth. Obviously, this is no longer the case. The nuclear family is no longer the core of the community, and nowadays, we live in fragmented, disconnected communities, far removed from nature, and often don't even know the names of our neighbors.

The vacuum of positive influences is then rapidly filled by popular culture, which focuses on sensationalism and entertainment value, not emotional, intellectual, or spiritual development—to the ultimate detriment of our children.

Furthermore, we live in a society that values capitalism and materialism above all else and judges a person's worth by the size of their bank account, not the size of their heart. These misplaced values then get displaced upon our children, further widening the feeling of being disconnected from their true nature: unconditional love and pure light, which have the power to heal absolutely anything.

Even the complex institution known as our healthcare system has become infiltrated with misplaced values. It is now driven by pharmaceutical and medical device companies, physicians, and surgeons trying to maximize their profit and hospitals that globally employ millions of staff and need to make a profit in order to remain viable. This perpetuates chronic disease, as costly treatments help fuel profits, and means that little emphasis is placed on either preventive medicine or true healing at a core level.

In fact, modern mainstream medicine has evolved hand in hand with pharmaceuticals and medical technology. When utilized in the correct context, these can be wonderful tools in treating and relieving the symptoms of chronic illness, but detrimental when viewed as an end in themselves and the patient's well-being no longer the sole focus.

What we are talking about here is the difference between living lives rooted in ego-based values as opposed to heart- or spirit-centered values. As discussed, this is the root cause of the problem of why so many people in modern society are chronically ill.

So how do we counter these dangerous trends in our current global paradigm, which not only threaten the health and life of individuals but of entire populations, the economies that rely on them, and humanity as a whole? This is the topic of the next chapter, which introduces the concept of bridging the two worlds that we live in.

KEY POINTS

- Healing is a process of unraveling the layers of illusion we have become accustomed to and identify with, in order to unveil our true nature.

CHAPTER 3

WALKING A FINE LINE

When we look at the majority of people, we find them locked in a struggle for survival, which is rooted in a fear of lack of abundance, a quality of the ego. The ego is the part of our being that interfaces with the physical world we live in and is essential for our survival. It is also the aspect of ourselves that perpetuates the fear-based false concept of our identity as physical beings living in a hostile universe.

When we see ourselves in this way, we feel that we are competing for limited resources and view others as adversaries, thereby replacing feelings of love, compassion, joy, and appreciation with feelings of apprehension, conflict, resentment, and turmoil. These feelings, if not transmuted, become lodged in our bodies, manifesting over time as anxiety and depression, which can eventually lead to chronic illness.

Not only do these negative emotions pollute our inner world and cause physical symptoms but they also result in the pollution of our outer world. This is reflected in the pillaging and plundering of our planet, resulting in environmental destruction of unimaginable proportions.

This is not just a problem of perception but one of misplaced identity. You see, our egos fear annihilation and, therefore, try to convince us that they are our true identity. Now, certainly our egos are an important aspect of our identity, but they are not the only aspect, and not even the main aspect, of who we are. Who we are is far greater than we can ever imagine.

Our appearance of being solid, physical beings is actually an illusion, as science tells us that the atoms of which we are composed are more than 99.99% empty space. If we break down atoms into their subatomic particles, we will find that they are just packets of energy vibrating at a certain frequency.

And what is energy? Energy is something that on the one hand defies description but on the other hand is known to all as the matrix of the uni-

30

verse. It takes many forms and can be manipulated and transmuted. This is what Einstein described in his famous mathematical statement, in which he equated energy to matter traveling at the speed of light squared.

So, essentially, all we truly are is a vibrational frequency or a resonant rhythm that can change density based on our inner state. Our inner state is influenced by our thoughts and feelings, and they, in turn, are often influenced by our outer life circumstances. This is how most people live their lives. But the majority of people have gotten it all wrong. We are not supposed to be the *effect* of our life circumstances; we are meant to be the *cause* of our life circumstances.

What this means is holding a high vibrational frequency, regardless of what is happening in our lives and transmuting those circumstances to match our inner state, instead of letting life circumstances transmute our inner state and decrease our vibrational frequency, with a resulting increased emotional density.

This book is going to show you how to do this.

We essentially have a foot in two worlds, but most of us do not realize this. We have a foot in the physical world of earthly existence with all its triumphs, defeats, and daily challenges and a foot in the spiritual world of our flawless and infinite pure essence. The problem is that most people identify with the former and not the latter, even though we are born into this world as pure vessels of light. As we progress through various life stages in our earthly existence, we accumulate layer upon layer of darkness, which obscures our essence as untainted beings of light. This is how we lose sight of our true nature and who we really are.

We may think that only adults are prone to this false identification, as the accumulated emotional density from a lifetime of experiences has led them away from their true nature. These days, though, children are becoming distracted by the numerous stimuli that are available for their entertainment and pleasure, from video games to social media to instant access to information on the internet, and have become lost in the sea of modern society and are succumbing to the dysfunction that has traditionally plagued adults.

Our challenge, as human beings on the earth, is to walk a fine line between the two aspects of our being. We have to acknowledge our physical existence, of course. We grow up in the world, establish careers, fall in love, have children, buy houses, pay the bills, get our hearts broken, plan vacations, watch movies, go to restaurants, get into fights with our family and co-workers, make up with them, fall down, get back up, and so on and so forth.

But we also have to acknowledge the deeper essence of who we are, which is timeless, flawless, infinite beings of light, beyond the limitations of our physical bodies—one with each other and with the Source, or as some call it, our Higher Power, Universal Intelligence, or the Divine Presence or God, which is the true nature of Ultimate Reality.

We have been placed here on this earth, with all of its vast experiences, both seemingly positive and negative, in order to create a frame of reference for us to know and experience who we truly are and merge with this Ultimate Reality. This is the one and only purpose of our existence on Earth; everything else is secondary.

Once we get a taste of what it feels like to merge with Ultimate Reality, all earthly experiences pale in comparison. The problem is that despite our true nature, we are all born as physical beings on the earth. We need to inhabit and traverse this physical plane at the same time as we are on the path toward realizing our true essence. But as we know, life on Earth can be quite daunting and overwhelming, and this takes us away from identifying with our true nature.

No one I have ever met is immune to this misalignment of identity. It can lead to the accumulation of layers of emotional density, as noted, and, if not dealt with, result in subconscious blocks and, eventually, chronic illness. But if we walk the fine line between this earthly realm and the inner realm of spirit, we can transmute this emotional density and use it as fuel for our higher consciousness.

The path I am suggesting does not involve denouncing the physical world, because the undeniable reality is that we are physical beings made of flesh, blood, bones, and organs. Instead, it is about living our lives in balance and not losing sight of our essential nature. This is the true meaning of healing in the highest sense. It is where the mystery of life resides.

KEY POINTS

- The secret to healing and reaching our full potential is to acknowledge the higher or spiritual aspects of our being and to harmonize this with our physical self.

CHAPTER 4

Opening to the Possibilities

Before we get to the actual path to healing, I would first like you to envision being completely healed of whatever you suffer from. The purpose of this exercise is to suspend whatever beliefs you have about the nature of your illness and imagine what is possible if you follow the path that I will be laying out for you.

It is important to envision your desired outcome, because this process occurs in your consciousness through a combination of pure thought and burning desire, and this must precede a manifest reality. Anything that you have ever acquired or achieved in your life was once a thought, which became an idea, which motivated action, which, if pursued with unswerving dedication, led to either your desired outcome or something that was equally desirable.

Okay, are you ready? Take a deep breath, and …

Imagine … being completely free of physical pain and discomfort.

Imagine … having no breathing difficulty.

Imagine … being the ideal weight.

Imagine … sleeping so restfully through the night that you are fully recharged come morning.

Imagine … being so full of vitality and energy that you are able to complete your work and your daily chores with grace and ease and still have the energy to do something that you enjoy.

Imagine … enjoying incredible sex.

Imagine … being able to reverse the aging process so you look much younger than your stated age.

Imagine … eating the healthiest food that is available and enjoying it immensely.

Imagine ... having a clear and worry-free mind.

Imagine ... being immune from the effects of stress in your life.

Imagine ... being able to reframe your limiting beliefs into empowering beliefs.

Imagine ... being able to transmute your emotional pain to fuel your higher consciousness.

Imagine ... living from your true essence and unleashing your creativity.

Imagine ... easily connecting with people you encounter in your daily travels.

Imagine ... all your personal relationships flourishing beyond your previous expectations.

Imagine ... being able to commune effortlessly with nature so that you become one with her.

Imagine ... being able to perceive beyond your five senses by honing your intuition.

Imagine ... being completely free of psychological fear.

Imagine ... always being in the flow.

Imagine ... being able to live your life's true mission sourced from your ultimate purpose.

Imagine ... being a source of peace and comfort to others who are in distress and suffering.

Imagine ... welcoming death, when it arrives, as a doorway to the next stage in your soul's evolution.

Imagine ... thriving in the face of uncertainty.

Imagine ... mastering the art of fulfillment and happiness.

Imagine ... emanating joy in everything you do and spreading it infectiously to others.

Imagine ... being a source of healing for humanity as a whole.

Imagine ... becoming one with the universe by realizing that your universe within is as vast and complex as the universe in which we exist.

Imagine ...

I don't want you to just read that list nonchalantly. That is why I wrote it the way I did. Slow down, and take your time reading it. I want you to truly envision and embody all these possibilities, even if you do not believe that they can be realized.

No matter what your health currently is and where you are in your life situation, nobody can take away your ability to exercise your imagination to visualize your highest dreams and aspirations in your mind's eye. Feel all the possibilities that I have mentioned in every cell of your body so deeply that no other outcome remains in your consciousness.

Remember that anything anyone has ever achieved was once a thought. It is when you focus on that thought so intensely that it permeates your consciousness that it has the potential to take form in the physical world.

Everything that I have previously mentioned, and more, is possible if you simply apply what you read in the pages that lie ahead with steadfast determination. So let's not delay. Let's begin on this incredible journey to the depths of your being to unveil your true nature and unleash your unlimited potential to heal!

KEY POINTS

- You must envision and embody the outcomes that you desire in your life in order to manifest them in your outer reality.

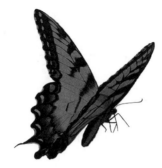

PART TWO

THE HEALING PROCESS
REVEALED AND EXPLAINED

CHAPTER 5

THE PATH TO HEALING

The insights gained from years of treating tens of thousands of patients for numerous conditions and my intensive study of the psychology of healing, consciousness, and metaphysics have led me to a process that I believe, if engaged in with unswerving conviction, can lead to the healing of any individual.

Again, I have to make the distinction between healing and cure. Healing does not necessarily equate to cure. Healing refers to realigning your entire being at all levels—physical, mental, emotional, vibrational, and spiritual, and existential—in order to create the optimal internal and external environment for your illness to be treated most effectively, with an improvement and, possibly, an elimination of your symptoms. I will go into this distinction in more detail in the next chapter.

The healing process has nine parts:

- Intention: Self and Universe
- Exploration
- Mentation
- Emotion
- Narration
- Vibration
- Motion
- Realization
- Creation

What modern medicine does is to compartmentalize our illness into an entity that is divorced from all other aspects of our lives, including our personal stories, thoughts, emotions, life circumstances, relationships, current and perceived stressors, and whether we are living out our true life's mission sourced from our true purpose. The nine-step process listed seeks to contextualize our illness within this greater framework, as noted above, in order to illuminate its root cause and potentially eliminate it once and for all.

It does not matter where you currently are in your life or what you are suffering from, this process can illuminate your true essence, which is pure, whole, infinite, already healed, and a guiding light for you and those whose lives you touch.

That's right, you're already healed, but this knowledge has become hidden from view over the course of your life. And no matter where your life has taken you up till this point, right here, right now, you're exactly where you need to be, otherwise you wouldn't be reading these words right now.

Before I start laying out each of these steps in more detail, I want to discuss the issue of research and the foundation of modern medicine, which is largely evidence-based.

Or is it?

Certainly, there are many interventions in current healthcare that have been proven to improve outcomes. Examples of these are the use of platelet inhibitors in myocardial infarction, early goal-directed resuscitation in septic shock, smoking cessation in patients with chronic obstructive pulmonary disease, to name just a few.

However, if you delve further into current medical practices, you will find that for every evidence-based treatment or intervention, there are numerous other treatments and interventions that have no valid evidence to show that they impact patient outcomes, namely mortality. Examples are cardiac catheterizations for patients with mild heart attacks (non-ST elevation myocardial infarction), chemotherapy for patients with various advanced cancers, and the use of vasopressors (medications that support the blood pressure) in patients with septic shock.

Despite the paucity of evidence that these interventions improve patient mortality, they are still utilized widely in the medical community. Why?

The reason is that even though patient mortality may not be affected, patients' symptoms are improved dramatically with these measures.

The point that I am trying to make is that, even though the process I have outlined above cannot be objectively studied, because the interventions and outcomes are difficult to measure, there are interventions in medicine that can be objectively measured that are still utilized despite not significantly impacting the main outcome of mortality, which is the focus of evidence-based medicine.

To proponents of evidence-based medicine who may be quick to discount the process I am introducing because the interventions cannot be objectively measured, I say, therefore: the benefits of such a process cannot be denied. Intuitively, we are aware of factors affecting our health that transcend our physical body. If this were not true then the condition known as takotsubo cardiomyopathy would not exist, as it is a strictly stress-induced cardiomyopathy acknowledged by cardiologists around the world, as mentioned earlier.

So, aspects of our being beyond the physical need to be engaged in order to effect comprehensive healing of any condition. This is what I am attempting to address with this nine-step process.

I do not discuss nutrition and exercise as stand-alone approaches; instead, I incorporate them into a greater framework of the healing process, since they are not effective as a sole means of achieving optimal health. There have been countless books written on nutrition and exercise, and knowledge of these modalities is readily available, and yet, we have a pandemic of chronic disease.

Therefore, it is not the lack of knowledge about diet and exercise that is the problem but something deeper and more visceral, namely how nutrition and exercise can support and enhance your inner state. If you can address your inner state effectively, then the outer aspects of your health will fall into place. After all, our outer circumstances are simply a reflection of our inner state. This is why it is important to align ourselves with our true nature, as the above process is designed to do.

Our true nature is who we are at our core when we strip away our thoughts, emotions, past experiences, personal stories, the roles we play, and our physical bodies.

When you contemplate this, what stirs within you?

If it is fear, then it is your ego that is feeling this, since its existence is rooted in all the things we need to strip away in order to reveal our true nature.

If what stirs within you is a sense of elation and freedom, then this is your true self or essence that is trying to emerge from the quagmire of all that you are not, everything that you once thought that you were.

If you are feeling a combination of fear and elation, then your current identity lies somewhere between ego and essence, and your job is to strip away all the ego structures that obscure and prevent your essence from emerging and revealing itself.

Hopefully, this book will start you on this incredible journey, the adventure of a lifetime!

KEY POINTS

- The healing process involves diving deeply into all the aspects of who we are including the physical, mental, emotional, vibrational, spiritual, and existential.

CHAPTER 6

THE NATURE OF THE PATH

I have mentioned on several occasions that there is a difference between healing and cure. This distinction is crucial because cure is an endpoint, whereas healing is a process.

In our goal-oriented, consumer-driven modern society, we often define fulfillment in our lives by specific endpoints. Examples include obtaining a car, a house, a university degree, a specific job, real estate, financial investments, a life partner, an ideal body weight, the perfect physique; the list goes on and on.

The problem is that although we define our fulfillment by certain endpoints, life itself cannot be defined this way, since it is a never-ending process that is continually evolving, moment by moment. Naturally, what we desire in life also evolves, and what was once a highly sought-after goal in the past may no longer be what we desire.

One may argue that everyone desires to be free of chronic disease, but we have to realize that our body, mind, and spirit are not static but dynamic entities that are also always evolving. This means that we may cure one condition but another may be right around the corner. We must always be engaged in the healing process and not just looking to cure a specific condition, since the healing process mirrors the process of life itself at all levels.

Even though the process I have outlined seems linear, healing is actually a nonlinear process that builds upon and reinforces itself with each cycle. In fact, it would be better demonstrated by a spiral, with the individual in question at the center of the spiral and each step represented by a turn of the spiral and building upon itself. Eventually, you end up where you started: embracing the unknown, which itself is a nonlinear concept that defies description.

I will discuss this specific issue in great detail in a future chapter. For the moment, though, the point I am trying to make is that, although I address the steps along the path to healing sequentially in this book, I believe that they must be engaged simultaneously.

For example, what often happens is that there is a flash of insight in which the individual is stripped bare of all that is not real, revealing her true nature. I believe this is the process one goes through when dying and in the phenomenon of spontaneous healing, which has been described in various accounts from all over the world. This can occur when the pain of suffering becomes so unbearable as to force the individual to dissociate from all his false identities, thereby unveiling his true nature.

Anita Morjani seems to allude to something similar in her landmark book *Dying To Be Me*. She describes how her true nature of unconditional love was revealed to her during her dying process. The truth is that she was undergoing a dying process; however, it was not the death of her physical body but the death of all that she identified with that is not real. She had to deteriorate to a point in her chronic illness in which her physical body was in danger in order to dissociate from all her false identities and have her true nature emerge. In essence, her near-physical death was a metaphor for the death of all her false identities, which is why I believe she reached this point in her illness.

I will say that this path is not for the faint of heart. It takes courage to cut through the illusions of false identity and get to the core essence of who you truly are.

In this earthly life, we become identified with numerous illusions, including our thoughts, emotions, family roles, professions, triumphs, defeats, emotional traumas, personal history, and so on. The reality is that we are none of these things; we are that pure unadulterated light that is the essence of our being and one with the entire universe. The problem is that most of us have become so layered with veils of illusion that it is difficult to see ourselves for who we truly are. Attempting to do so often results in retaliation from our ego in the form of a fear response, which is why this path is so challenging for most.

The ego wants us to identify with falsehood because it fears its own annihilation. However, this path is not about annihilating the ego but of merging the ego with our true nature, which is sourced from our Higher Self. When we do this, then all the aspects of ourselves which we once identified with, such as our thoughts, our emotions, and personal history, all come into greater perspective and fuel our journey toward our true nature, which is one of pure being or consciousness.

There are two types of fear: actual fear and psychological fear. Actual fear is fear as a result of real danger, such as an encounter with a jaguar in the Amazon jungle. Psychological fear is a false fear, which is created by our ego in order to keep us in our old patterns, which are often dysfunctional and meant to keep us from changing, which is threatening to the ego. This is the reason why people often remain stuck in old and outdated patterns of thinking and behaviors, despite a conscious realization that a change in these would result in more joy, peace, and happiness.

It is inevitable that on the path of healing, we will encounter psychological fear. This is especially true when it comes to embracing the unknown. This fear must be confronted with unswerving conviction if we are to progress on this journey. It represents a threshold that all on the path encounter and must be viewed as a sign that we are on the right path rather than a deterrent. The process of confronting and overcoming psychological fear will be addressed as we discuss the different steps along the path of healing. I have also devoted an entire chapter to the topic of overcoming fear.

One of the most powerful ways to facilitate change in anyone or in any situation is to ask the right questions. Asking the right questions can be transformational and dramatically change the course of your life. At the end of each of the following chapters on the steps to the path to healing, I provide a set of questions that can be used by healthcare and healing practitioners as diagnostic and therapeutic tools to help their patients and clients go deeper within to get to the roots of what ails them. These questions can also be used as tools for self reflection and your own deeper inquiry.

As you go through the steps on this journey, I encourage you to journal about your experience. Journaling is a powerful tool. It can help declutter your mind, organize your thoughts and feelings, and facilitate your progress on the healing path. So let's not delay any further. Let's start the journey!

KEY POINTS

- The healing process is not a linear process but is more like a spiral, with each step of the process defined as a turn on the spiral.
- The spiral of the healing process often collapses in on itself in the phenomenon of spontaneous healing.

- To engage in the healing process requires courage as psychological fear can arise at each step of the process.
- Psychological fear must be confronted at each stage of the healing process with unswerving conviction to reveal its illusory nature, which is created by the ego.

CHAPTER 7

INTENTION – SETTING THE STAGE

The fact that there are people who do not want to be healed may be a shock to some of you but not to someone like myself, who has treated tens of thousands of patients over the course of the last 18 years.

The reality is that there are those who may feign an interest in being healed but actually want to remain sick. They are not committed to healing in the core of their being.

I have encountered many reasons why someone may not want to be healed, including:

- Being chronically ill may allow the individual to get attention they desperately desire and cannot get any other way.
- Illness may convey a sense of identity on the individual that they cannot get any other way, especially if their true nature has become obscured by layers of emotional distress and trauma.
- The individual may have become so used to being ill that they do not know any other way of being, and this has become their so-called "normal state."
- They may experience guilt associated with healing in situations where close family members are also chronically ill.
- They may hold false beliefs that, as we age, we are all meant to eventually become sick.
- They may have unrecognized subconscious blocks and limiting beliefs that state that it is impossible to heal.

Anybody who is stuck in the paradigm of their chronic illness and has no desire to heal likely has some subconscious blocks to healing. At this stage, it is not important to remove these blocks; it is only important to realize that they are likely present.

If you have read this far, then you likely realize that you have some subconscious blocks to healing. These blocks will be addressed later on, but it is not necessary to dissolve the blocks to make the decision to want to be healed. What is necessary is to declare your intention to heal, both to yourself and to the universe. Declaring your intention to heal to yourself helps ground this desire deep within, so it can take root and grow over time. Declaring your intention to heal to the universe tests your conviction and garners its support on your journey. Let's look at each of these in more detail.

SELF

So how does one cross the invisible threshold from wanting to remain stuck in the paradigm of chronic illness to wanting to be healed?

This usually involves two issues: lack of meaning in one's life and the illusion of separation, hence the lack of connection to others. At the intersection of intention, meaning or purpose, and connection lies inspiration. Inspiration is the first step needed in order to cross the threshold to the healing path.

Let's first address lack of meaning.

Meaning is crucial if an individual wants to be healed from chronic disease. Meaning is the essence of life; it is your powerful "why." Your powerful why is the driving force that motivates you to get up in the morning. If you do not perceive any meaning in what you spend the majority of your day doing, this means that you do not have a powerful why. You are not living; you are slowly dying.

It is no secret that most people hate their jobs and do them only to support their families and pay their bills. It is also no secret that many people are unhappy in their marriages and other personal relationships and only remain in them for the false sense of security and fear of loneliness. I believe that both situations result from a lack of meaning in one's life.

The problem is that if you are not guided by a greater purpose or mission, which is what meaning is, you end up settling for any substitute you can find for true meaning to anchor your life.

Often these anchors become a job or a relationship or both, but if they are not sourced from true meaning, then they will not fill the void in your life. This leads to more discontent and unhappiness, which fuels destructive behaviors, such as watching hours of television, overeating, drinking excess alcohol, smoking, using illicit drugs, and an endless array of false pleasures that take the place of a meaningful job or relationship.

Destructive behaviors like these, along with the negative emotions that fuel them, create a platform for physical symptoms to emerge, eventually leading to chronic illness. It is no wonder that chronic disease has become a pandemic in modern society.

Meaning is closely tied to purpose or life mission; therefore, the way to find the path to healing from chronic illness is to find your powerful why.

Why do you get up in the morning? Is it to simply go through the daily motions of sleeping, getting up, having breakfast, going to work, coming home, having dinner, watching television, or surfing the internet and sleeping again? If this is what your life has come down to, then you have not found your powerful why, which is tied to your life mission.

But how does someone find their life mission when they are stuck in the quagmire of modern society, which keeps us locked in a struggle for survival, doing meaningless work, and seems to want to distract us from what matters?

Our distractions range from television, movies, and video games to numbing ourselves with senseless addictions such as tobacco, alcohol, and narcotics in order to deal with the increasing demands of our complex daily lives. These distractions may provide a temporary escape from our mundane, stressful daily lives, but they only keep us from discovering our life's true mission.

I would like to make a distinction between life's purpose and mission. Our purpose is to fully awaken to our true nature and be a conduit for something greater than ourselves to express itself through us. This "something greater" will have a different name for different individuals, groups, and cultures and can be referred to in a number of ways such as Higher Power, Ultimate Reality, the Universe, Source, Being, Consciousness, Unconditional Love, or simply God. Our mission is to express our purpose in our own unique way based on our unique gifts, skills, aptitude, and experience.

We can ask a number of questions to discover our life's mission.

- One question is, what were you fascinated with as a child that kept you busy for hours? Think back to those carefree, endless days when pursuing your childhood passion was all that mattered in your life.

- Another question is, what do you enjoy doing as an adult that keeps you so mesmerized that you lose track of time while engaging in it?
- What talents and abilities do others complement you on?
- If time and money were not issues, how would you want to spend each day?
- What draws your attention when you are not distracted by the activities of daily living?
- What brings joy, love, and peace to your life?
- Which people do you admire for their qualities, pursuits, and accomplishments?
- Who did you dream of becoming when you were a child?

These are just some of the questions you can ask yourself to get on the path to pursuing your life's mission. Furthermore, you can use your personal life story to gain insight into your life's unique mission. I will explain this in more detail in an upcoming chapter on the narration step of the healing process.

It may seem like a tall order to discover your life mission and pursue this path, but this does not have to be an overwhelming endeavor, take you away from your current livelihood, or create more burdens in your life.

You can simply start by spending five minutes a day contemplating the questions I have mentioned above and using these as a starting point to explore your inner world and find what lies within. This can be done in silent meditation before your day begins, on your drive to work, during your lunch hour, during an afternoon break, on your drive home from work, or in the evening when all is still and quiet and there are no distractions.

There are absolutely no excuses for anyone to not be able to come up with five minutes a day for this pursuit, as there is nobody who does not spend at least five minutes on their commute to work engaging in senseless gossip and idle conversation, watching television that does nothing but numb the senses, playing video games that do the same, writing or reading mundane posts on social media, and a host of other mind-numbing daily activities. Even if you don't partake in any such activities, you can easily give up five minutes of sleep to engage in silent contemplation on the questions that can lead you to your life's mission.

Your life's mission or your powerful why does not have to be on a massive scale, such as ending world hunger or ending global regional conflict. It can be as simple as raising your children with the utmost compassion and presence; deciding to start your own backyard garden in order to supply your family, friends, and neighbors with fresh, homegrown vegetables to help promote the overall health of members of your community; volunteering at a local seniors' center to provide companionship to the elderly; or committing to performing one act of kindness every day, such as smiling at a stranger.

The multitude of ways in which your life's purpose can be expressed is like a rainbow that contains the full spectrum of colors but is actually just pure light before the process of refraction breaks it up into its distinct parts. Each of us is needed to express our own unique mission in this world in order to create a harmonious symphony of collective expression, analogous to pure unrefracted light.

The metaphor of pure light and the rainbow also contains another meaning. If we view the individual colors of the rainbow in isolation, each one is limited in how much it can illuminate whatever it shines on. But if we combine them, they create a radiant light that can illuminate anything in its path. Humans are analogous to the different colors of the rainbow, in that they cannot live in isolation from each other; they need to connect in order to fulfill their potential.

This brings us to the second issue preventing people from wanting to be healed: the illusion of separation and our lack of connection, closely tied to lack of meaning.

You see, your mission is not a solo project to be carried out in solitude but must contribute to the greater good of humanity and, ultimately, the greater good of the planet. It is because you have been living in isolation from your family, your friends, your neighbors, your immediate community, and the global community that you have lost the sense of any meaning in your life.

As you begin to reconnect with others, you will start to notice the needs of society—first at a local community level, then at a global level. This helps plant the seeds of compassion in the soil of your consciousness, which grows the tree of positive action, which allows you to reap the fruits of service. Therefore, the key to finding meaning and your mission is to reconnect with yourself, others, nature, and the planet.

So how do we even start to end the illusion of separation and reconnect with the greater whole?

You can simply start by paying attention. Pay attention to the world within you and the world around you. I don't mean the almost numb, diluted attention you use during your commute to work in rush hour traffic, listening to mindless radio with only enough awareness to avoid hitting the car ahead of you as you navigate stop-and-go traffic. I mean the deep, focused attention you need in order to truly recognize the subtleties in the world around you—the type of attention that someone you are listening to feels completely healed by. And if you don't believe that it is possible to heal someone simply by listening deeply to them, then you have never listened to anyone at a deep enough level to experience this.

As you begin to pay attention to the world within, you start to illuminate your thoughts and emotions and journey farther into your true nature. I will discuss this in more detail in future chapters, when I delve into the concept of inner flow. As you begin to pay more attention to the world around you, your senses start to open up and inform you about your world in such a comprehensive way that you may begin to notice things before your senses have fully comprehended the nature of the situation. This is what is referred to as intuition.

This kind of profound attention can be practiced in your regular daily routine, while driving to work, while interacting with co-workers, while talking with customers or clients over the phone, and while eating your lunch as you savor every morsel of food that enters your mouth. It can also be cultivated at the end of the day, when you greet your spouse and your kids and spend the last few hours of the day in their presence.

Although deep attention can be practiced in any situation, I do recommend a practice to help shift your awareness: spending time in nature fully attentive to your surroundings for as much time as you can spend. This is a practice that has been cultivated in history by indigenous cultures around the world and is known as the "sit spot." The purpose of the sit spot is to connect deeply with nature, which was, at one time, intimately tied to the survival of individuals and entire tribes. After all, nature is the source for the essentials of survival: fire, water, food, and shelter.

For your purposes, spending time in nature with this kind of keen attention will, over time, help to hone your senses and heighten your sense of intuition. It will also reinforce your connection to something greater than yourself, thereby helping to end the illusion of separation and reestablish a sense of meaning and purpose in your life. This can help rekindle and ignite your life's mission and give you a reason to want to be healed.

Once you have begun to uncover the deeper meaning of your life and illuminated the illusion of separation from which you have suffered, you then need to announce your intention to heal to yourself. The way to set and announce your intention to yourself can vary. What follows is a sample intention statement, which you can play with and modify as you see fit:

> *My intention is to fully heal myself of (name your condition).*
> *I have suffered with this condition for too long, and it is time for me to let go of it once and for all. I realize that my life has a greater purpose here on this earth and my condition is impeding me from fulfilling my life's mission. My condition keeps me from fully experiencing my connection to others and to the greater whole of which I am a part, which is another reason I must relinquish this condition for good. My life's mission has direct bearing on my connection to the greater whole, because this mission is for the greater good of humanity and the planet. This is why I am willing to do whatever it takes to fully heal myself of my condition and to realize my greater potential, free of this condition.*

In conclusion, in order to cross the invisible threshold from not wanting to be healed to wanting to be healed, you must find your powerful why, which will lead to cultivating your unique life's mission. You must also end your illusion of separation from the greater whole by reconnecting with others. This can be accomplished through carrying out your life's mission, which is always tied to the greater good of humanity. You can also do this by reconnecting with nature by spending more time with her in contemplative meditation.

UNIVERSE

We have talked about intention as it relates to self in the previous section. Once your intention to yourself is established, then comes the next step, which is announcing your intention to the universe.

By announcing your intention to heal to the universe, you declare where your attention and focus lies, which fuels and illuminates your journey on the healing path.

This is probably the most crucial step in this journey, because once you announce your intention to the universe, it will test your conviction to this path. All sorts of obstacles will arise to deter you. You will start to come up with excuses, and tasks will pile up all around you that interfere with your healing journey. Your illness may seem to get worse, and the path to healing will start to look daunting and near impossible to traverse, and you will start to wonder why you ever thought you could heal in the first place. It is at this point that you may give up on this journey and fall back into old patterns of victimization by being enslaved to your chronic disease.

So why does this happen? Is the universe there to discourage you? Are you forever bound to your current self-induced prison with no hope of ever escaping? Is there no point in even trying to pursue a lofty goal, such as trying to heal your chronic illness?

Fortunately, none of these statements is true. What is true is that courage is required to walk the path to healing, and the universe rises to test your courage once you announce to it your intention. It does this to ensure that you will be committed to this path once you take the first step, not because it wants you to fail but because it wants to bear witness to your conviction to this path. This is why the things you want most in life often seem to be the most difficult to achieve. Fear arises, and courage must be cultivated in order to surmount this fear.

Courage arises in those whose conviction about wanting to be healed surpasses their willingness to accept the continued suffering that accompanies living with chronic disease. Therefore, the purpose of announcing your intention to heal to the universe is to raise the necessary courage to walk the healing journey with unswerving conviction.

If you have established meaning and connection in your life through your intention to yourself, it becomes easier to cultivate this courage to keep yourself committed to your healing journey. This highlights an important point regarding the entire healing journey: no step lies in isolation; they are intricately connected.

This creates a continuum, as opposed to separate individual steps or a sequential process to follow. This continuum reinforces the oneness of all things and highlights your connection not only to yourself but to the whole. It is only in relation to the whole that a context of healing can be created, since the need for healing is relative.

In the absolute sense healing is not needed, because in your original, pure essence, no illness can exist; however, in the relative world, of which you are an integral part, the essence of who you are in its purest form becomes lost through your experiences in the relative. Your announcement to the universe of your intention to heal is not only a call to courage but a proclamation that you still have an inkling of knowledge of your true essence. This connects you to the source of all that exists, which serves as a guiding light on your journey.

The way you show your conviction to the universe is through your thoughts and words. You must think thoughts of being healed, regardless of what your present circumstances are. This is difficult to do for many people, because for the most part our minds ruminate over countless negative thoughts. *I am not good enough. What can go wrong will go wrong. I will never amount to anything. I will never get the raise. My spouse and I never get along. Things can only get* worse. *I will never get out of debt. Life is a struggle. It's a dog-eat-dog world. Only the strongest survive. I am one more day closer to death. What's the point of even trying? She will never go out with me. I hate Mondays. The world is doomed. Love hurts. Everybody is selfish. Nobody cares. I will never heal.*

You get the picture.

Negative thinking has become a pandemic in modern society. It has many origins, including our upbringing, challenges we have faced, the media that constantly bombard us with bad news, unsupportive peer groups, past failures and rejections, and these are just the tip of the iceberg.

Negative thinking is usually hardwired in us from our early childhood, which makes it difficult to counteract. This is the reason negative habits such as smoking, alcohol abuse, and consuming too much sugar are hard to break. These same negative thoughts are often the catalysts for chronic disease and usually originate in the limiting beliefs that we have all been programmed with. I will discuss the link between limiting beliefs and chronic disease and how to eliminate them in a subsequent chapter. At this point it is simply enough to recognize how limiting beliefs and their consequences have become ingrained into our nature.

The way to start to counteract the tsunami of negative thoughts is by starting with one positive thought and reinforcing that thought at every moment you can. That thought could be: *I am perfect health, I am unconditional love, I am unlimited abundance, I am the highest intuition,* or *I am radiant joy.*

The purpose of starting with this one positive thought is not to remove the wave of negative thinking with which we are bombarded every day (this will be discussed in a subsequent chapter of this book as part of another step in the healing process); instead, it is to show the universe what you believe is actually possible for you.

Once you do this, it will initiate a wave of support for your journey from places that you never even imagined. Thought has the power to do this because thought is nothing but pure energy, and energy attracts like energy. It is not enough to simply think the positive thought but to believe it with every fiber of your being. Even though the ultimate goal of the healing process is to go to a place beyond thought, this is where it must start, because thought is a dominant aspect of our daily lives.

The second way to show the universe your commitment to healing is through the medium of language—your words. Language is the primary verbal way we communicate with each other and must be in line with your thoughts if you are to heal. Language is the verbal expression of your thoughts, which originate in your mind and are witnessed by your consciousness.

When we examine language in general, we find that most of our language is simply an expression of the negative thoughts that predominate in our minds in modern society. Most people do not fully appreciate how powerful the medium of language is, and it is only those who use direct communication in their daily lives or who are public speakers who truly appreciate its power.

All you have to do is witness master speakers in action, such as a Tony Robbins or Oprah Winfrey, to realize the power of language. The difference between them and you is that they have an audience of thousands, whereas your only audience is your own mind, which bears witness to the words you speak.

This is why it is so vitally important to choose your words wisely. Words and phrases that are repeated constantly eventually become embedded in your subconscious mind, especially at a young age. This is why it is crucial to speak words of kindness, compassion, enthusiasm, encouragement, and love to your newborns, infants, and children.

Your language is always a direct expression of your state of mind and announces your intentions to the universe. Just like you would not want someone else to speak harsh or cruel words to you, you should not be speaking similar words to yourself. Your words should always express your highest intention, which is to heal.

There are two aspects to using words to express your highest intention to the universe. The first is to pay full attention to the words that come out of your mouth in any situation. This is often difficult to do, since it is usually our subconscious mind that is doing the speaking, and our words are often reactionary and not well thought out.

This will become easier once you illuminate your subconscious mind, which I will discuss further on. In the meantime it is simply enough to realize that your words are a direct expression of your thoughts, and if you can start to reinforce a positive healing thought in your mind, as discussed above, it will directly affect the language you use.

Another way to know what you are going to say before it becomes manifest is to use a "gatekeeper," which checks your words at the door of your mind before they exit your mouth.

I use a simple technique called a breath pause. Before I am about to speak, I breathe out fully and hold my breath until my body tells me that I need to breathe. What this does is gives me a few seconds to think about what I am about to say before I say it and to determine if it will be constructive or destructive to the situation at hand. You can develop your own gatekeeper to keep your words in check before they are even spoken. Obviously, there are times when you need to verbally react to a situation immediately, such as when someone is in danger, so using your gatekeeper may not always be practical; however, it can be used in most situations, such as when you are simply engaged in daily conversation.

The second aspect of using words to express your highest intention to the universe is something I call a "declaration." This involves repeating a healing mantra on a regular basis until it becomes a regular part of your daily rituals which may include prayer, meditation, and exercise.

This may sound similar to an affirmation, but an affirmation is an announcement to your subconscious mind with the intention of reprogramming it over time, whereas a declaration is your announcement to the universe of your highest intention.

Formulate this as an "I am" or "I create" statement not an "I want" statement. That's because "I want" will always leave you in a state of wanting, whereas "I am" or "I create" is a declaration of what you already are and just need to experience in your physical reality.

I will give you an example of a simple mantra I use daily that announces to the universe where I am heading in my life: "I create and expand my love, abundance, success, happiness, power, flow, influence, and time each and every day." You don't have to use my mantra; just create your own, based on your own intentions for your healing. The important thing is to have a mantra that becomes part of your daily morning rituals.

In conclusion, it is vitally important to announce your intention to heal to the universe by being mindful of your thoughts and words, reinforcing positive thoughts in your mind, using only positive language, and speaking a healing mantra on a regular basis.

KEY POINTS

- Setting your intention is the first step in engaging the path to healing.
- Setting your intention to heal has two components, the first of which is to find your powerful why and to find your unique life's mission.
- The second component to setting your intention is to end your illusion of separation and realize your connection to others, your immediate environment, nature and, ultimately, the universe.
- It is important to announce to the universe your intention to heal through your thoughts and words.
- You must replace your negative thinking with positive thinking by starting out with a single uplifting thought and reinforcing it as often as possible throughout the day.
- You must also pay attention to the language you use on a regular basis and ensure that it reflects the highest truth about yourself and not the illusion of who you once thought you were.
- You should have a personalized healing mantra that you repeat to yourself on a regular basis.

QUESTIONS TO ASK YOUR CLIENTS

- Have you ever set the intention to heal?
- If you did, were you able to follow through on your intention?
- If you were able to follow through on your intention, what was the outcome?
- If you were not able to follow through on your intention to heal, what do you think kept you from following through?
- What were your childhood dreams and ambitions?
- What have you enjoyed in the past or enjoy doing currently that keeps you so thoroughly engaged that you lose all track of time?
- What are your natural talents and abilities that you can perform effortlessly and that others complement you on?
- What brings joy, love, and peace to your life?
- Who are the people who you admire for their qualities, pursuits, and accomplishments?
- If you knew you could not fail, what would you attempt to do?
- What are some ways in which you could embody your connection to other people, nature, the earth, and the universe?
- What are the negative thoughts that sabotage your thinking?
- What are some positive thoughts that you could replace your negative thoughts with?
- How have your words hurt you or someone you care about?
- Has this experience helped you realize the power of your words?
- What words can you use to to encourage the people you care about?
- What is a universal healing mantra that you could use on a daily basis as a declaration to yourself and to the universe of your highest intention?

CHAPTER 8

Exploration –
Dancing with the Void

The next step in the healing journey is probably the one that is most difficult to do: exploring and embracing the unknown.

The unknown is a subject that typically evokes fear and trepidation, yet is a constant throughout life, from birth onwards, when we are thrust headfirst into the unknown.

Life's unknowns begin around the time of our birth. Modern technology such as ultrasounds and amniocentesis may give some idea of the baby's health, but a lot of unknowns still remain. These include natural factors that could affect the health of the baby, including the mother's nutrition and overall health, stresses that the mother is under, plus a multitude of complications that we hope never will but could occur at the time of birth: preterm labor, prolonged labor, abnormal presentation, premature rupture of the membranes, umbilical cord prolapse or compression, and amniotic fluid embolism, to name just a few.

After birth, the number of unknowns multiply exponentially, including when will your baby start to crawl, talk, walk, leave diapers, learn to socialize, be ready for preschool, sleep independently, and lose his or her fear of the dark?

As your baby enters childhood and adolescence, the unknowns multiply further and include how will your child perform in school, will they socialize well with peers, will they be good at sports, will they fall into the wrong crowd, will they experiment with drugs, will they want to go to college or university, will they be able to establish a successful career, will they meet the partner of their dreams? These questions are just the tip of the iceberg.

I have been talking about external unknowns, but there are even greater internal unknowns. Medical science claims to know how the human body works, but we scarcely understand anything. Sure, we know the gross workings of the human body in the areas of anatomy and physiology, and we even understand the cellular and molecular mechanisms of how our bodies function. Despite this, there are many unknowns when it comes to our bodies and how they work.

One example is why are human beings the only living things that exhibit consciousness, and at what point in our development does this consciousness enter our bodies? What is the mechanism by which our bodies age and eventually deteriorate, leading to death? How do cells truly communicate important information to each other, such as when the body is being attacked by invading pathogens? How does our brain hold the vast amount of information we absorb from birth through to our elder years, and how are we able to retrieve this information at will?

Then there are the existential unknowns. When was the universe born? If the universe has a starting point, what existed before it? Is the universe infinite? If it is not, then what lies beyond its borders? Do other dimensions or parallel universes exist? What is the nature of God? What happens after we die? One of the greatest unknowns is that our inner world, namely our bodies down to the subatomic level, our thoughts, emotions, and consciousness are as vast and complex as the universe itself.

The point I am trying to make is that we live with the unknown at every step of our lives, yet we fear it more than anything else. This fear is unwarranted. How can we fear something that is our constant companion throughout our lives and an integral part of who we are?

We have the illusion of solidity, but quantum mechanics tells us that our subatomic particles are actually more than 99.99% empty space and mainly consist of different vibrational frequencies of energy. Yet our world appears solid—our bodies, the ground, trees, mountains, animals, cars, houses, buildings, and the numerous other objects in our world. The fact that everything appears solid yet is more than 99.99% empty space defies description and is one of the greatest mysteries of life. And what is mystery but the human mind seeking to understand the unknown.

This means that our bodies also have the illusion of solidity yet are mainly empty space at the subatomic level. What is this empty space, which comprises the majority of who we truly are? Science can help point us in the right direction, but it cannot answer this question. This is the reason why the creation of the universe remains a mystery to this date. Science claims that the universe arose from the "big bang," the rapid expansion of matter from a state of extremely high density and temperature; however, science cannot explain what initiated this cataclysmic event.

Science also cannot currently explain what existed before the big bang and the creation of the universe. Since the reality that arose out of the big bang is more than 99.99% empty space, the implication is that before the big bang, there was simply this empty space. This implies that there was and is an invisible field out of which all we perceive as real arose, and it is this invisible field that is our true nature. If we truly are this invisible field, then can we shape and morph our physical reality?

The way to answer this question is to scrutinize what shapes our outcomes in daily life, from our health, wealth, and relationships to our personal time and freedom. Do these outcomes not simply come down to the choices we make?

For example, if we choose to smoke cigarettes, drink alcohol to excess, eat a lot of sugar, breads, and pastries, and sit in front of the television or play video games in all of our free time, what outcome could we expect? It is only logical to imagine that we would become overweight, develop hypertension, glucose intolerance, leading to diabetes, heart disease, and possibly a stroke. Even if we did not start out with these conditions, making the choices I indicated earlier would certainly lead to these outcomes.

On the other hand, if we were to quit smoking, stop drinking alcohol to excess, eat more green vegetables, legumes, nuts, seeds, berries, and lean protein and use our free time to engage in moderate exercise, what outcome would we then expect? We would likely be full of energy, sleep better throughout the night, be happier, able to complete our daily tasks with vigor and on time, have better sex and have some free time to do the things we love.

What makes the difference in the outcomes in these two cases? Choice. It seems like a fairly simple concept, but it all comes down to this one thing that we do in every moment of our waking lives—make choices.

Choice is therefore the driving force that directs our invisible field to mold the reality we experience in our physical lives on this earth.

Once we realize that we have the power to direct this invisible field, which compromises most of who we are, through the choices we make, we can begin to cultivate a different relationship with the unknown. The unknown then becomes a field of possibility rather than something that induces fear and anxiety. This field of possibility becomes a venue for exploration that becomes engaged when we push the edges of our comfort zone.

You may ask how this is relevant to healing illness.

Whether it is a progressively deteriorating chronic disease or an acute illness, when you become sick you are immediately thrust into the realm of uncertainty as your symptoms progress. Symptoms are an unpleasant sensation that are experienced in the body and perceived by the mind. Uncertainty arises when we wonder how to deal with these sensations and prevent them from getting worse.

Many people seek conventional treatments that fall into the realms of medications, procedures, and surgery. There is nothing wrong with seeking these treatments because this is what we have been taught to do through the conditioning of the modern healthcare system. It is natural to seek to relieve the symptoms of the illnesses we suffer from.

The problem is that we only seek external solutions and fear entering inner space because, for most of us, it remains an unexplored realm. Our parents, schools, religious institutions, and others involved in our education have not taught us that all our answers lie within, including how to heal, and anything that remains unexplored remains unknown. This is why we have not cultivated any inner approaches to healing our illnesses.

I mentioned earlier that choice is the hidden force that directs the invisible field to mold our reality. We simply have to make the choice to explore the unknown to find answers to our healing. This exploration begins in the hidden recesses of our inner realms. We will likely be more comfortable sticking to what we know and not going within, but this is what keeps us stuck in the paradigm of living with chronic disease rather than healing.

Once we make the choice to explore our inner world to seek answers to our healing, we are embracing the more than 99.99 percent of our reality that is empty space, or the invisible field. This is the start of a transformational process at all levels, including body, mind, and spirit, and it is done simply through the power of choice.

We can start to get comfortable with the unknown by exercising the power of choice on a regular basis to gently nudge us out of our comfort zones. I usually talk about using choice to *lean* outside your comfort zone, instead of *stepping* outside your comfort zone. It may sound like semantics, but the reason I suggest using this language is that, to the ego, leaning outside your comfort zone will seem less intimidating than actually stepping outside it. As you lean outside your comfort zone more often, you will eventually be able to step outside it fully over time.

There are many ways you can lean outside your comfort zone. Health-wise, you can start to eat healthier foods, such as more green vegetables, legumes, seeds, nuts, and berries, push the limits of your exercise capacity, and try new and exciting forms of physical activity, such as rock climbing, windsurfing, or skiing.

In the realm of your relationships, you can start smiling at strangers more, try to strike up a conversation with someone you don't know or just met, reconnect with estranged friends and family members, and choose to be more kind, loving, and compassionate to your life partner.

In the realm of your career, you can engage your boss and co-workers in creating innovative solutions to problems at work, do extra training to learn new skills, and even go back to college or university to further your education. Even more powerful are the inner choices you can make that enrich your mind, your heart, and your soul. You have already made such a choice by choosing to read this book.

As noted earlier, we often get stuck in the realm of our inner world because this remains largely an unexplored territory. In addition, several aspects of our inner realms need to be navigated effectively in order to tap into the wealth that lies within us, including our subconscious mind, our limiting beliefs, and our unresolved emotions. This is where our journey will take us in the following chapters.

KEY POINTS

- The unknown is our constant companion at every stage of our lives and, therefore, does not need to be feared.
- You can engage the unknown through the medium of choice.
- You should make choices that force you to lean outside your comfort zone. This is how you grow and transform and, ultimately, heal.

QUESTIONS TO ASK YOUR CLIENTS

- What choices have you made or continue to make that keep you stuck in your comfort zone?

- How have these choices directed or limited your experience of life?
- What is the worst possible outcome if you were to lean outside your comfort zone?
- Could this worse possible outcome hurt or harm you in any permanent way?
- What one simple thing could you do right now to lean outside your comfort zone?

CHAPTER 9

Mentation –
Clearing Your Subconscious
Blocks and Limiting Beliefs

Mentation refers to all the psychological issues that keep us from healing. These usually revolve around the subconscious mind, one of the most challenging aspects of healing.

The subconscious mind controls most of our beliefs, behaviors, thoughts, habits, and actions and thus drives the majority of our experience of life. When we scrutinize our daily routines, we start to see where the subconscious mind operates.

One of the first things most people do when they wake up is to go to the bathroom to relieve themselves. This is an example of a subconscious behavior, because it does not require any conscious thought to perform but is something we do naturally. Another example of a subconscious behavior is the route we take to drive to our place of work if we have been at the same workplace for any significant period of time. This is usually well ingrained in us, and making this daily sojourn requires little or no thought.

Now let's contrast this with a conscious behavior. Let's suppose that your usual route to work is disrupted because of a major accident and has been blocked off for several hours. In this case, you still have to get to work, but you have to think about which alternative route you will take to get there. This requires using the conscious mind, since the new route must be discovered by you and is not part of your usual routine.

As you can surmise, subconscious behaviors become such through repetition and reinforcement. This is why our usual driving route becomes so natural to us that we do not have to think about it. Unfortunately, not all of our subconscious behaviors are beneficial to us.

An example of this is smoking. Smoking often starts out as a fad when we are young and feel invincible. We may see our friends and peers engaging in this behavior, and in our quest to fit in and be accepted, we are led to do the same. Smoking may start out as a fun and seemingly harmless activity that we engage in with our friends. Over time, however, it becomes a reinforced behavior that we seemingly cannot control because it has been taken over by the subconscious mind. This is why it is so difficult to quit, and no amount of motivation or willpower can put an end to this nasty habit, and people who consciously try to quit smoking often do so for a time but eventually relapse.

Motivation and willpower are sourced from the conscious mind and are not powerful enough to override the programming of our subconscious mind that drives us to smoke. This is true of any pathologic behavior, such as abusing alcohol or illicit substances, watching excess television, surfing the internet aimlessly with no purpose in mind, and overeating, to name just a few. This is how addictions are born and why they are so difficult to overcome.

I have so far discussed actions that are sourced from our subconscious mind, which can adversely affect our health if they result in unhealthy habits leading to addictions. However, if we dive further into our subconscious mind, we discover more sinister ways in which it can undermine our health, by generating negative thoughts and limiting beliefs.

We all know what negative thinking is, since there is not one person I know who has not been a victim of this at some point in their lives. But what are limiting beliefs?

A belief is a thought that we accept as being true, even though it may have no proof of its validity in actual reality. An example of this is a belief in unseen forces that guide us in our earthly life, such as angels. I am not debating the existence of such beings. We may believe that angels exist, and we may even feel their presence in our daily lives, but there is no objective way to prove the validity of this belief. We can point to miraculous events we may have experienced at the hands of angels, but there is still no objective way to prove their existence. It therefore follows that limiting beliefs are those thoughts that we accept as being true that prevent us from reaching our true potential. If we look at the majority of people, we will find that we suffer from literally hundreds of limiting beliefs. Unfortunately, these limiting beliefs determine not only our experience of life but our ultimate potential.

One limiting belief is that as we age, we are bound to develop chronic disease. We may have grown up around sick grandparents, which reinforced this limiting belief.

Another limiting belief is that our physicians know what is best for us and should be obeyed without question. I consider this a limiting belief because, although most physicians usually have accumulated a wealth of knowledge about treating disease, they know very little about promoting health, good nutrition, and preventing disease, as these subjects are not taught in medical school. What is taught is a reactionary approach to treating acute illness and chronic disease when they arise.

Another limiting belief is that the only treatments for diseases, once they arise, are medications, procedures, and surgeries. Most doctors have little or no knowledge of more holistic healing practices, many of which have been practiced for thousands of years before the advent of modern medicine, and this can tremendously impact the course of an acute or chronic illness. This does not mean that patients may not need medications and surgery, but offering these and not including counseling, good nutrition, exercise, the benefits of natural and herbal remedies, spending time in nature, and meditation can only limit the patients' potential to overcome their illnesses.

We have only touched on a few of the limiting beliefs that can affect health, but they can also pervade other aspects of our lives, such as relationships, finances, our ability to experience true freedom in our lives, and our ultimate happiness. But where and how do these limiting beliefs arise?

Subconscious actions, such as driving to work, are usually the result of repetition. However, limiting beliefs are usually more deeply embedded in our psyche and have roots that often go back to our childhood and early infancy. When we are first born into this world, we are free of any positive or negative experiences. Because our minds are empty vessels, they take in our environment and condition our thoughts into creating our beliefs about life.

For example, if you experienced physical abuse as an infant or child, you will grow up with a belief that people are to be feared because they are all out to hurt you. Although, this may be true in certain cases, it is not true of the majority of people but, because of your experience of abuse, it will condition your subconscious mind to keep you on the defensive and to never trust anybody.

If, as a child, you witnessed your parents fighting about finances, you will grow up with a limiting belief that money is scarce and any substantial amount can only be acquired through struggle. This will affect the level of financial success you achieve in your life, regardless of your means of earning an income.

Similarly if you grow up seeing your parents and grandparents with chronic health issues, you will be conditioned to believe that this is the norm and is inevitable for you. Alternatively, you may rebel against such an outcome and decide that you will do everything in your power to avoid chronic health issues, but this is not usually the case for most people.

So if our limiting beliefs arise out of our early childhood experiences and subsequent conditioning, how are we to combat them to avoid stunting our potential in all aspects of our lives, including our health?

The first step in reframing our limiting beliefs is to interrupt their patterns and to realize that they are simply beliefs with no basis in truth or reality. For example, if our grandparents or parents have suffered from chronic disease, does it mean that we will suffer the same fate? There is absolutely no basis in reality for this belief, as chronic disease is the end result of many factors beyond genetics, including diet, level of exercise, self-defeating habits such as smoking, exposure to environmental toxins, and negative social environments, to name just a few of the influences on our health. Therefore, we must realize our limiting beliefs as simply beliefs and not facts.

The next step is to become conscious of where our limiting beliefs have derailed us from the outcomes we desire, such as freedom from illness, not having to take medications, achieving excellent health, and living with boundless energy.

Once we can visualize our desired outcomes, this helps put our limiting beliefs into context. We realize that they have simply been deterring us from our desired outcomes.

Once we become conscious of how our limiting beliefs have kept us from our goals, we now need to find examples of where our limiting beliefs are not true. To use the example I introduced earlier, if you believe that you are destined to suffer the same health fate as your parents, to counter this, you can look to many examples where children do not suffer from the same illnesses that their parents do. In fact, you may not even have any signs of disease but only believe that you eventually will because of heredity. Therefore, you may be your own proof that you can be free of whatever fate has befallen your parents.

The next step is to find an alternative meaning to your limiting belief. For example, seeing your parents suffering from chronic illness may not be a sign that you are destined to suffer the same fate but that you should take better care of your health to avoid the same fate.

The next step is to eliminate your limiting beliefs and to replace them with empowering ones. In order to understand how to eliminate our limiting beliefs, it is helpful to use an analogy.

Our psyche can be likened to a storage room in our basement. It is often the least visited room in the house because it is simply used for storage and we only go there when we need to retrieve something or store further items. Because it is rarely frequented, unwanted guests can take residence in the storage room, such as spiders, centipedes, cockroaches, and other bugs that live underground. The storage room can also accumulate a lot of dust and filth, because it is rarely cleaned on a regular basis. In the same way, if our psyche and subconscious mind are not attended to on a regular basis, unwanted guests such as subconscious blocks and limiting beliefs can become established and take residence there.

Now, in order to eliminate spiders, centipedes, and other bugs from the storage room, we must turn on the light or shine a flashlight into that room to find them first. Once we do this, we find that they scurry and try to hide in order to more deeply embed their presence in that space. It may take multiple attempts with the light source to find and remove these persistent pests.

In the same way, our subconscious mind must also be illuminated in order to uncover our subconscious blocks and limiting beliefs and eliminate these entities. Once these limiting beliefs are identified, it is not enough to simply remove them. They must be replaced with empowering beliefs.

So what are our limiting beliefs around health and chronic disease? We have already mentioned a few, but here are some of the more common limiting beliefs that plague many of us.

I will never heal. I will always remain sick. Medications are the only treatment for my disease. I must always live with my disease. I should never question my doctor because he always knows what's best for me.

Chronic disease is a normal part of aging. My disease is a punishment for the bad things I've done. I'm genetically programmed to have chronic disease. Disease can only be treated from the outside in. I have no control over my health. I am powerless in the face of my illness. Spontaneous healing is not possible.

So what is the process of rewriting our limiting beliefs? When I talked about finding bugs in the storage room, I discussed shining a bright light into the room to identify the bugs so they can be removed. In the same way, we must illuminate the subconscious blocks and limiting beliefs in our psyche. This can be done through a simple meditative process that I will describe as follows.

Find a quiet place, either indoors or outside in nature, where you will not be disturbed for at least twenty to thirty minutes. You can keep your eyes closed or open, whatever is comfortable to you.

The key to this meditation is to visualize light flooding your body from all directions—from above, from below, and from all sides and angles. Imagine this light flooding every cell of your body and illuminating these cells fully, so that they become tiny points of light. Imagine these points of light coalescing into a larger field of light that consumes every aspect of your physical self.

Once you can visualize yourself as a brilliant being of pure light, say the limiting belief you want to reframe and eliminate from your psyche. For example, you could say, "All the places where I believe I will never heal and always remain sick, I erase and eliminate this belief from every aspect of my being."

Then proceed to replace this limiting belief with an empowering belief. Using the example above, you could say, "I am fully healed from my chronic condition." You can repeat this process for any limiting belief that you suffer from.

Let's go through each of the limiting beliefs I have mentioned above, one at a time.

- "Everywhere I believe that I will always remain sick, I erase and eliminate this belief from every aspect of my being. I overcome my illness fully and completely."

- "Everywhere I believe that medications are the only treatment for my disease, I erase and eliminate this belief from every aspect of my being. Medications are only one part of my treatment, and part of a more holistic approach that heals me fully."
- "Everywhere I believe that I must always live with chronic disease, I erase and eliminate this belief from every aspect of my being. I live with no chronic disease in any part of my body."
- "Everywhere I believe that I should never question my physician because he always knows what is best for me, I erase and eliminate this belief from every aspect of my being. I accept my physician's advice regarding my health and put this advice into context with my entire whole health healing plan."
- "Everywhere I believe that my disease is a punishment for the bad things I've done, I erase and eliminate this belief from every aspect of my being. My disease has nothing to do with punishment but is simply something my body is experiencing because of my lack of understanding and scrutiny of my inner world and how this is reflected in my outer health."
- "Everywhere I believe that I'm genetically programmed to have chronic disease, I erase and eliminate this belief from every aspect of my being. Genes are only part of the story of chronic illness and manifest in the context of environmental influences that affect their expression."
- "Everywhere I believe that disease can only be treated from the outside in, I erase and eliminate this belief from every aspect of my being. Disease is optimally treated from the inside out."
- "Everywhere I believe that I have no control over my health, I erase and eliminate this belief from every aspect of my being. I have full control over my health."
- "Everywhere I believe that I am powerless in the face of my illness, I erase and eliminate this belief from every aspect of my being. My illness is powerless in the face of the full extent of my presence."
- "Everywhere I believe that spontaneous healing is not possible, I erase and eliminate this belief from every aspect of my being. Spontaneous healing not only is possible but has been

a proven phenomenon in, literally, thousands of cases and probably many more that are unknown to the general public."

The next step, after rewriting a limiting belief into an empowering belief, is to embody this belief. This is done by finding evidence that your new belief could actually turn out to be the truth and then taking immediate action on your empowering belief.

For example, if your limiting belief was that you can only be treated for your illness with medications, look for examples of individuals who have come off or decreased the doses of their medications through making lifestyle changes around sleep, nutrition, and exercise. I have many examples of patients who have been able to do just that.

If your limiting belief was that your medical doctor is the only source of knowledge and wisdom to treat and heal your illness, look for examples of individuals who have supplemented their primary treatment with integrative, holistic, and mind-body approaches to healing. If you scrutinize the cancer community, you will find many patients who integrate their chemotherapy and radiation therapy with more holistic approaches, as described by Dr. Kelly Turner in her landmark book, *Radical Remission: Surviving Cancer Against All Odds.*

If your limiting belief was that you have no control over your health, look for examples in your life where you were able to take ownership of what ails you and were able to facilitate the process of healing.

For example, if you were a child and fell off your bike and scraped and cut your knees, you may remember your mother helping you clean the dirt off the wound, cleaning it with antiseptic solution, and putting a band aid or dressing on the wound. This is an example of taking ownership of a medical condition and taking action to facilitate the process of healing.

For any limiting belief that you have held around your health, you can eliminate this, create an empowering belief, and find living proof of the truth of this belief if you do enough research. This forms the basis of taking immediate action on that empowering belief.

The process of eliminating and replacing limiting beliefs is not a one-time process and needs to be repeated over and over again. Just like the bugs that can easily return to the storage room after they are removed, subconscious blocks and limiting beliefs can persist after one clearing. This is why the meditation described above needs to be repeated over and over again for every limiting belief we can identify. Once your limiting beliefs have been removed and replaced with empowering beliefs and embodied with living proof of their validity, you will start to clear a pathway to journey to your inner world where the source of your healing truly lies. Just like removing debris from a road, your path will be cleared for you to take the next step.

As you proceed along this inner journey you will come across the next obstacle to healing in your path: unresolved emotions. This is the subject of the next chapter.

KEY POINTS

- The subconscious mind controls most of our beliefs, behaviors, thoughts, habits, and actions and thus drives the majority of our experience of life.
- Limiting beliefs are those thoughts that we accept as being true, even though they have no proof of their validity in actual reality, which prevent us from reaching our true potential.
- We all suffer from limiting beliefs, which can be identified through negative thought patterns and recurrent personal challenges that regularly confront us.
- Limiting beliefs can be identified, seen for their falsehood, reframed into empowering beliefs, and embodied into a new manifest reality.

QUESTIONS TO ASK YOUR CLIENTS

- Can you identify your limiting beliefs through your negative thought patterns and personal challenges? Make a list of them.
- Ask yourself if these limiting beliefs hold any validity.
- Can you find evidence to prove that your limiting beliefs are not true?
- Can you find an alternate meaning to your limiting beliefs?
- Can you reframe your limiting beliefs into empowering beliefs?
- How can you embody your newly formed empowering beliefs?

CHAPTER 10

Emotion – Burning Through Your Unresolved Feelings

Emotions are one of the most complex entities to explain in words. They are how the mind communicates with your Higher Self and are felt directly in the body.

For example, if you are walking down the street and a stranger approaches you and asks for your wallet, you will feel fear. Immediately, signals are sent to your brain, and your hypothalamus is alerted to signal your autonomic nervous system, which activates your sympathetic nervous system.

The sympathetic nervous system prepares your body to deal with the danger by increasing your heart rate, and hence your cardiac output to increase oxygen delivery to your skeletal muscles. It also constricts the blood vessels to your internal organs, such as those of your digestive system, which are not needed to deal with the immediate threat. Your pupils also dilate to enhance your vision during the threat.

The sympathetic nervous system also stimulates the adrenal glands to release cortisol, epinephrine, and norepinephrine into the circulation. This results in the "fight-or-flight" response, which is manifested by an increase in heart rate, dilatation of the bronchial airways, and an increase in the metabolic rate, which helps you to respond effectively to whatever is threatening you. This example shows how emotions, fear in this case, are experienced in the body.

But what are emotions? What role do they play in our lives?

Emotions are the language of the soul. They are experienced in the physical body, because the body is the vehicle through which our souls experience life on Earth.

Because we have such a wide range of experiences in our earthly lives, we have a wide range of emotions we can feel. Often these emotions are not distinct but form a spectrum, much like how pure light can be refracted into different wavelengths of colors after passing through droplets of rain. Our emotions can range from utter despair and desolation to unbridled ecstasy, and everything in-between.

Emotions are what give our life experiences meaning, but they are very subjective and are not an absolute. For example, you may perceive the loss of your job as devastating because it was the only source of your income. However, if you take a step back and put this into perspective, you will start to realize that your job was not fulfilling, you did not get along with your boss, and were anxious the entire time you were at work. So although you lost the only source of your income, it was probably the best thing that could have happened to you because it was not what you were born to do and was sucking the life out of you. This loss freed up your time to pursue your true passion and discover your life's mission.

You can see how our emotions are subjective. So even though emotions are what give our life experiences meaning, it is important to note that it is the meaning we ascribe to these experiences that is subjective. The problem arises when we take these emotions as an absolute truth and fail to look for the deeper significance of the experiences that generated them.

What follows from this is that there is no such thing as a negative emotion. What, you say? Did I hear that right? Yes you did. Let me repeat that profound truth. There never has been and never will be such a thing as a negative emotion.

So how can such emotions such as sadness, grief, despair, depression, shame, regret, anger, hatred, jealousy, rage, and fear be perceived as anything but negative? I will try to shed some light on this issue.

They key here is that our emotions are our soul's experience of life situations felt in the body. If what we experience is perceived as negative, then it simply means that we have a false sense of being incomplete or lacking something. This happens as a result of how we interpret events in our lives. But our souls can never be incomplete or lacking, because they are whole and complete by nature.

For example, if an intimate relationship suddenly comes to an end, we may feel sad because we feel a loss of love. But this is a false perception because love is our soul's true nature, so it is something we can never lose. We simply perceive a loss of love because our soul experiences union with another soul in the physical plane through the medium of a relationship. This is a relative experience, with the absolute truth being that your true nature is that of unconditional love. I will delve more deeply into this in an upcoming chapter.

So if this is true, why do we feel sad when a relationship ends? It is because we have not yet realized our true essence as love, so the feeling is necessary to alert us that there is something greater that we have yet to understand or realize about ourselves. In fact, this is the purpose of all of our emotions.

Another example is the emotion of anger, which is usually experienced when something unexpected happens to us or something we are expecting to happen does not happen.

The truth of the matter is that there is nothing that can happen to us that we did not intend at a higher level of being. We only experience unexpected events as such due to a lack of insight into our multidimensional nature and our highest levels of intention. On the flipside, when we feel joy, peace, compassion, or ecstasy, it is a confirmation and a celebration of who we truly are.

The problem arises when we interpret our emotions as an absolute truth and not a reminder of where we lack understanding or an affirmation of our true nature. This usually happens when we have an emotionally intense experience that makes us feel uncomfortable. In these situations, we often suppress those emotions because of how they make us feel.

For example, if you were physically abused as a child you probably felt fear, rage, and despair. If you felt that you could do nothing to prevent the abuse, you would eventually learn to suppress those emotions and put up with the abuse. The problem with this approach is that the emotions are suppressed but do not dissipate. They will settle and embed themselves in your physical body, and you will experience them as all sorts of physical symptoms, which, over time, will evolve into disease.

Now, to use the earlier example of an abused child, if that child grew up suppressing those feelings of fear, rage, and despair, they will become internalized. What happens in this case is that if the same individual faces a situation that even remotely resembles the abuse faced in the past, these emotions will resurface and they will be reminded of the abuse endured as a child.

For example, let's say that the abused child is now in adolescence and is bullied at school. Even if the bullying is not as physically or emotionally traumatic as the childhood abuse, those childhood emotions will be triggered because they were suppressed and internalized and lay dormant until a sentinel event, in this case bullying, causes them to resurface. If those emotions do resurface, they will again be suppressed in order to avoid the pain that they cause and the past pain that is brought to light.

Eckhart Tolle has named this phenomenon the "pain-body" in his landmark book, *The Power of Now*. Even if these unresolved emotions, or the pain-body, are not triggered for some time, they can, over time, result in chronic stress and anxiety, which can evolve into physical symptoms and, eventually, chronic disease. So in our efforts to avoid the angst caused by the pain-body, suffering can be prolonged.

How do negative emotions translate into chronic disease?

If we do not allow ourselves to fully experience so-called negative emotions because they are too painful, they become suppressed. These suppressed emotions result in chronic stress, which causes the same physiologic response as imminent danger. This means that suppressed emotions stimulate the adrenal glands to secrete cortisol. Cortisol, when secreted in the face of an actual threat or imminent danger, helps the body deal with the acute situation, through the fight-or-flight response. It also suppresses the immune system, which is involved in the inflammatory response. This is why it has an anti-inflammatory effect. However, as I have mentioned already, suppressed emotions result in chronic stress, which overstimulates the adrenal glands. This overstimulation results in a decrease in cortisol secretion over time and, therefore, a decrease in cortisol's anti-inflammatory effect. Without cortisol, inflammation is free to run rampant throughout the body, which is one of the main factors leading to chronic disease.

Now let's go back to my earlier proclamation that there are no negative emotions.

Emotions are the language of the soul that are experienced in the body. So let's look at the same example of the abused child who feels fear, rage, and despair. What is the soul trying to communicate in this situation?

The soul or Higher Self is trying to communicate to the child those aspects of herself that need to be loved, namely the aspects that feel the fear, rage, and despair. This is in order for the individual to realize her true soul nature as love. The question then arises, how can a child be expected to navigate those feelings and realize their true purpose?

In an ideal world, the child would not be faced with the situation of abuse. She would only grow up experiencing love from everyone she encounters, which would reinforce her true nature as love. But we live in a less than ideal world, and children often experience things that make us angry and lose hope in humanity.

Now, most children express their emotions freely without reservation. Think of a six-month-old baby who has soiled his diaper and feels uncomfortable. He will continue to cry until he gets the attention of his mother and she realizes that he needs to be changed. In this situation, the baby is relatively sure that his expression or emotion will get him the attention he needs in that moment.

The situation is entirely different for the abused child whose cries often go unheard. In this case, it seems natural for the child to suppress her emotions to avoid the pain she feels. Furthermore, there is no way for her to know that her unresolved emotions will result in suffering over time, leading to anxiety, depression, and chronic disease. In fact, I'm sure that every one of you knows someone who is suffering because of unresolved emotions or the pain-body. Even if the individual has had no known traumatic experiences in their lifetime, they are likely to have experienced some level of birth trauma, as a result of leaving the mother's womb and descending via the narrow birth canal in order to enter this world.

In the mother's womb, we are safe, secure, nourished, and comforted. When we enter this physical world at the time of birth, we are being thrust into a completely new and strange environment that we have not yet experienced and where we do not have the same safety, security, and reassurance we had in the womb. This is a universally traumatic experience for all, even if there are no complications at the time of birth.

Often these unresolved emotions are not the result of something that the individual has experienced in their lifetime. There is also the issue of ancestral trauma, which I will explain here.

Human history from the time of the crusades to modern-day political turmoil and terrorism is chock full of stories of ongoing pain and anguish inflicted on one group or culture of individuals from another group or culture. The intense emotions surrounding the accompanying suffering often go unresolved, not only in the lifetime of those individuals who are the victims but also through subsequent generations. This so-called "ancestral trauma" gets passed on through the generations to present-day individuals who feel the pain and suffering, but have no idea why they feel this way. The intense feelings associated with this ancestral trauma often go unrecognized and unresolved and can result in physical symptoms and chronic illness over time.

So how does one deal with unresolved emotions related to trauma from their lifetime and beyond?

I am going to describe an exercise that will help you deal with your unresolved emotions. The first step is to discover what your unresolved emotions are and their source. I have already mentioned that these emotions can be triggered by current events that mimic the original source of those emotions. So the first step is to recognize when, recently, you were triggered. Think back to recent times when you felt very intense and uncomfortable emotions and try to identify the cause or trigger for those.

Once you have done this, the next step is to go back farther in time and identify an earlier incident when you felt similarly intense and uncomfortable emotions and again identify their trigger. Keep repeating this process until you are able to trace a thread back over time through these emotional outbreaks and their sources.

Try to find a pattern and go as far back in time as possible. The goal is to trace this thread back to the original source of the pain-body that keeps getting triggered. Once you are able to identify this original source, you need to find a time and place where you will not be disturbed for a good period of time, at least one hour.

When you are in this time and place, you need to set the intention that you will release the emotion that has held you prisoner for so long. Make sure you are in a safe and comfortable place where you will not be disturbed, either indoors or outside in nature. You can either close your eyes or keep them open, if you desire.

Now recall the original event or cause fully in your mind, and experience the emotions around it as completely as possible. Now, I realize that in most cases, these have been emotionally traumatic events, and it would seem irresponsible to ask someone to re-experience the emotions around them. The truth of the matter is that as long as the situation that caused the pain-body in the first place is no longer an active situation, it cannot harm you. You think it can harm you because of the pain-body you have built up around the past issue and all of the suffering that accompanies it. However, in reality, as long as the issue is not active, the unresolved emotions will only cause the perception of danger but not actual danger.

If the situation in question is still active and ongoing, then you should not be doing this exercise. You first need to end or remove yourself from the situation before you can heal the emotions around it. If you suffer from suicidal depression, you should consult your mental health specialist before undertaking this exercise.

If you do this process and go back to the sentinel event that led to intense and painful emotions and birthed the pain-body, you don't need to re-experience that event. What you need to do is to feel the emotions around it that you have suppressed.

Feel them as fully as you can. Let the waves of grief, sorrow, despair, anger, fear, and desperation wash over you, like the waves of an ocean. Feel them as intensely as you can, right to their core. Do not resist them any longer. You may find yourself crying uncontrollably as you unleash years of pent-up grief. You may find yourself screaming incessantly as you release years of pent-up rage. Just let the process unfold naturally, as you relive those suppressed feelings. What you will find, if you let yourself feel these emotions to their core, is that you will eventually reach a place of indescribable peace.

The hurricane is a great metaphor for your emotions, because at their center is a profound peace much like the calm one finds in the eye of a hurricane. Once you have born the wrath and fury of the hurricane and are able to reach this place of deep inner peace, you know that you have healed the pain-body, which has become fuel for your consciousness to shine brighter. The emotions that created your pain-body can no longer hold you hostage like they did in the past, as you have fully released them.

If, as a result of doing the earlier exercises, you have been able to identify more than one incident from your past that has fueled your pain-body, you need to repeat this process for each of those incidents until you have released all the emotions that surround them.

What about smaller incidents that we face on a daily basis that also feed our pain-body, such as being cut-off while driving to work, an argument with your spouse, dealing with a creditor, or an argument with your boss, to name a few? You can repeat the same process for each of the unresolved emotions that arise from daily minor issues on a regular basis. In fact, you may find it useful to do this emotional releasing exercise several times a month or even once per week once you have cleared your major unresolved emotions.

What if you have a recurrent negative emotional pattern but cannot identify the sentinel event that led to this pattern because it has been repressed for a long time or is the result of ancestral trauma, which is not always apparent?

In this case, you do not necessarily have to identify the sentinel event that led to the recurrent negative emotional pattern. What you have to do is to identify where the emotion is felt in the body.

For example, sadness and despair are often felt as a tightness in the chest or in the heart region. Anger is often felt as a throbbing in the head. Once you are able to identify the part of your body where the emotion is felt, you can then be present with the emotion and feel it fully, right to its core, as long it takes. You may have to repeat this process several times to fully release the emotion and reach a place of deep inner peace.

The truth is that we experience emotions in every moment of our lives, and the key to living fully is to allow ourselves to experience these emotions fully, even if they are painful. It is the painful emotions that, if not felt fully and repressed, can lead to suffering, symptoms in the body and, eventually, chronic disease. Emotions are part of the full spectrum of human experience and must be allowed to percolate through us unabated if they are to reveal to us the deeper meaning of our lives.

Our life experiences form a narrative that represents the journey of our soul in the physical realm, and our emotions are how our mind and body communicate with our Higher Self or our soul. It is only by experiencing the full range of human emotion that we can begin to glimpse our true nature because all emotions lead us back to unconditional love.

The purpose of emotions, no matter where they land on the spectrum, is to reveal our true soul nature to us, which is why they all must be experienced fully. That is what is meant by the phrase, "Live your life to the fullest." It does not mean accumulating more consumer goods, more life experiences, or more friends and acquaintances; it is about being completely present to what you are feeling in the immediate moment and letting it pass through you relentlessly. This is how your soul experiences your life in the physical realm and what ultimately reveals your true nature to you.

Emotions often arise out of various experiences in our lives, and the accumulation of all our life experiences form a narrative or life story. If we don't handle our emotions, they can obscure the underlying message or meaning in our narrative and can lead to identification with our various life stories, which removes us farther from our true nature.

They can also obscure the lessons that our narrative is meant to reveal to us about why we are here in this earthly existence and our greater life's mission. This leads us into two upcoming chapters, which will discuss unraveling the stories around our illness and finding the deeper meaning behind our life stories.

But before we get to these issues, in the next chapter, I would like to delve more deeply into one of the most crippling emotions we all deal with on a regular basis: fear.

KEY POINTS

- Emotions are the soul's expression of our experience of our earthly life, and are experienced in the physical body.
- There is no such thing as a negative emotion, since it simply points to a lack of understanding of our true nature.
- Unresolved emotions can be triggered by experiences similar to the sentinel event that led to the unresolved emotion in the first place.
- Unresolved emotions, if not processed and experienced fully, can lead to physical symptoms and chronic disease.
- The full spectrum of human emotion needs to be experienced in order to reveal to us our deeper spiritual nature of unconditional love.

QUESTIONS TO ASK YOUR CLIENTS

- What are the recurrent emotional patterns in your life that keep you stuck and keep you from reaching your full potential?
- Can you trace a recurrent emotional pattern back to the sentinel event that birthed it?
- If you cannot trace a recurrent emotional pattern back to the sentinel event, where do you feel these emotions in your body?
- If you were to experience the emotions around the sentinel event

to their fullest extent, what is the worst thing that could happen to you?

- How would your life transform if you were able to burn through your unresolved emotions fully and experience the peace that lies at their core?
- What is keeping you from burning through your unresolved emotions and releasing them once and for all?

CHAPTER 11

Overcoming Fear

Fear is one of the most fascinating and crippling human emotions. All of us, at one time or another, have been overcome with fear.

As I have mentioned earlier, there are two kinds of fear: actual fear and psychological fear.

Actual fear involves a true danger, one that is often life threatening. An example of this is if a masked criminal holds you up at gunpoint in a dark alley in the slums of the city in which you live. In this case, there is a legitimate threat to your life, and the fear is warranted. Psychological fear, however, is a misperceived danger or threat in a situation in which there is none.

An example of this is coming to work on a Monday morning and being completely ignored by your boss as he walks by you in the hallway outside your office. Most people would ascribe all sorts of meaning to such an event, with no evidence of any truth behind their interpretation.

For example, you may think that your boss is upset with something you did or your recent performance at work. This could evolve into worry and stress over where you went wrong. This could lead to fear of potentially losing your job which could lead to the fear of how you will support your family and pay your bills. You will then begin dwelling on how you will ever find another job and what you now have to do to prove your worth to another employer. This may lead to a change in your behavior at work with your colleagues and the boss who snubbed you, which could create an issue where none ever existed.

Now, there is a possibility that all you believe about this event is true. However, if your performance at work to that point has been exemplary, and your boss and colleagues have previously been pleased with you, it is unlikely that any of your fears are warranted.

Another possible interpretation of this event is that your boss is so preoccupied with another issue that has nothing to do with you that he failed to notice you as he walked by you. He may be preoccupied with a personal issue at home, another employee, a difficult client, last quarter profits, a new product launch, a new direction that the business is taking, or any number of issues that have nothing to do with you. But because our minds have a tendency to misinterpret events before they have all the facts, the situation is interpreted in a way that creates unwarranted fear, which can lead to chronic stress and, eventually, illness. I call this psychological fear because it is created by the mind and is not an actual danger or threat.

Other situations in which we feel psychological fear is when we aspire to goals that we're not sure we can achieve. A classic example is that you want to ask someone out on a date but are afraid of being rejected. Another example is asking your boss for a salary increase. In both cases, you have a goal in mind, but before you even know what the outcome will be your mind has created fear around this goal.

The truth of the matter is that it is natural to feel such psychological fear because it is often a learned response from situations in our early childhood and youth in which we may not have always gotten what we desired. Our ego latches onto these memories and reinforces our fears. It does this in order to keep us safe from rejection and disappointment because the ego's role, in our evolution, has been to help us survive.

The problem with this is that even though our ego has been integral to our survival, it often keeps us from taking the necessary steps to achieve great things in our lives. The problem is not the feeling of psychological fear but what we do with the feeling. If we dwell on psychological fear and let it pollute our thoughts and affect our daily routine, it will eventually lead to chronic stress and illness, as I have already mentioned. What we need to realize is that psychological fear is usually a threshold that we have to face on the path to our goals and ambitions, a gate that we must pass through in order to achieve these.

Fear usually arises out of some sort of risk, and there are many kinds of risk we can face. In physical risk, there is a threat to your physical body and well-being. An example of this is mountain climbing or skydiving, where there is a potential risk to life.

Emotional risk usually involves our dealings with other people and our relationships. An example of this is telling someone you care deeply about that you love them. The risk here is that the feelings will not be reciprocated.

Intellectual risk involves seeking to learn and apply a new body of knowledge or skill.

Spiritual risk can take several forms. One type of spiritual risk is when you go against your religious upbringing and choose a different religious or spiritual path. The risk here is that you will be shunned and condemned by your parents, siblings, and extended family members. Another type of spiritual risk is trusting in a Higher Power. The risk here is that the existence of a Higher Power cannot be rationally proven and is based solely on faith or belief. There is the potential that your beliefs in a Higher Power are not true.

Existential risk involves beginning to question the reasons behind the creation of the universe and your own very existence. The risk here is that you could create a crisis of identity and meaning that could dramatically alter the current course of your life situation.

I would like to give you a rational approach to dealing with any fear that you may experience in your life, actual or psychological. But no matter what is causing the fear you are experiencing, action is always a must. This will become more clear as I discuss the steps to dealing with any fear that you face.

The first step is to assess the situation: the source of the fear. Is there an actual threat or danger to your life? If this is the case, then you are dealing with an actual fear, and you must take any immediate action possible to remove yourself from the source of the threat or danger. For example, if you are being confronted by an armed gunman, you either give him what he wants, so that he will leave you alone, or you go along with his demands until you can find an opening in the situation to escape.

If there is no actual threat or danger, you must then ask yourself, what is the source of my psychological fear? It may be that you are imagining the worst possible outcome of the situation.

For example, in the case of asking out an attractive person on a date, your mind may fear the potential outcome of rejection. The problem is that your mind is imagining the worst possible outcome from a spectrum of potential outcomes. One possible outcome could be that they agree to go out with you. Another possible outcome is that they do not become a love interest but a friend who you can spend time with. Another possible outcome is that they are not romantically interested in you but by going through the process of asking them out, you gain the courage to ask out someone else.

Our minds have a tendency to latch onto the worst possible outcome and make this a reality before the actual situation has a chance to unfold naturally. The way to deal with this is to let your mind experience the emotional outcome of the worst possible situation.

For example, in the case of asking out an attractive person on a date, let your mind experience rejection and feel this outcome fully. Then ask your mind, what is the worst possible thing that could happen? Will you die? Of course not! Will you be embarrassed? Potentially. Will your ego or your pride be temporarily bruised from this rejection? Possibly, but this is not the end of the world. You will, eventually, get over this rejection and realize that there are many other people you could potentially date.

What you are doing here is putting the worst possible outcome into perspective and realizing that the emotional fallout from this outcome is probably not as bad as your mind may have imagined it. You are also telling your mind that the worst possible outcome is only one out of a spectrum of other possible outcomes, many of which may be desirable. The issue at hand is that you will never know the eventual outcome if you do not take action on the issue that causes the psychological fear.

What this means is that psychological fear is not an insurmountable obstacle that you should retreat from but a threshold that you need to cross if you are to grow and evolve.

Think about it. Some of our greatest accomplishments have been achieved despite our fears about taking action. When a baby is first learning to walk, they hesitate, stumble many times, and may even get hurt while trying. But the baby does not give up and keeps on trying despite their fear until they are finally able to walk with full balance.

This is how we should handle our psychological fears. As long as there is no imminent threat to our lives, we need to move toward our fears and through them. This is the only way we will achieve the spectrum of desirable outcomes that can come out of the situation. It is where real inner growth and wisdom occurs. This is why fear is a signpost on your journey that guides you to the greatest possibilities for your life.

The other thing to realize is that courage is not the absence of fear but the ability to do what needs to be done in spite of fear. If you give in to the fear, then you are allowing your ego to dictate the course of your life, which thinks it is keeping you safe from disappointment. If you move toward and through your fear, then you are living from the highest aspect of who you are, namely your consciousness, being, or spirit, which cannot be threatened by anything. Fear is simply your Higher Self calling you to live the greatest version of who you are in order to open yourself up to experience the best possible outcome in any situation. So feel the fear, and do it anyway!

KEY POINTS

- There are two kinds of fear: actual fear and psychological fear.
- Actual fear indicates a real and imminent threat to your life.
- Psychological fear is a perceived or contrived threat created by your mind where one does not actually exist.
- Psychological fear is a threshold we must all cross in order to realize the greatest possible outcomes for our lives and to grow and evolve in wisdom.

QUESTIONS TO ASK YOUR CLIENTS

- Can you recall some milestones in your life where you felt fear?
- Did you take action despite the fear?
- If you did, what was the outcome?
- If you didn't, what possible outcomes did you deprive yourself of?
- What in your life currently causes you fear?
- What is this fear telling you about the direction you must take?
- What could be the greatest possible outcome from making the choice that is causing you fear?

CHAPTER 12

Narration Part 1 – Unraveling the Story Around Your Illness

Narration refers to the stories we create around our illnesses. These stories are usually tied in with identity and tend to arise because we identify so strongly with our disease processes. This perpetuates the chronic disease and prevents us from healing.

Stories that patients use to perpetuate their disease process are many and various. We will examine a few of them in this chapter.

One of the most common stories may be that of victimization, feeling like you are a victim of whatever ails you. Where does this sense of victimization come from? It usually arises when we feel helpless and powerless in the face of a chronic disease as a result of limiting beliefs and unresolved emotions, as discussed in previous chapters.

Once the scaffolding of subconscious blocks and unresolved emotions is dismantled, the story of victimization is no longer valid and usually falls away without much resistance. However, for some people, stories of victimization are so ingrained they do not come apart so easily.

How do you know if you have a victimization story around your illness? Clues are that you feel sorry for yourself; you find yourself talking about your disease with everyone you know, including family friends and even acquaintances; you look to your physicians and specialists to "save" you; you do not question why you are ill but just accept it blindly; you feel that you have no control over your chronic disease; you take no initiative to learn about your disease; and you find yourself embracing your disease like a long-lost friend.

What is the root of the victimization story? It lies in a loss of identity. When you lose sight of your true nature, this creates a void that needs to be filled. You try to fill this void with food, alcohol, drugs, internet, television, sex, parties, or any other experience you can get your hands on. Chronic disease can also creep in to fill this void, and often does, after you have exhausted all other void-fillers. The problem (or perhaps attraction) with chronic disease is the constant companionship it offers. It all too easily fills the void arising from not identifying with our true nature.

So how do you unravel the victimization story around your illness? By seeing it for the falsehood it is. This becomes easier to do once you have cleared your limiting beliefs and unresolved emotions. Then all you have to do is to see this story for the falsehood it is. Victimhood is simply an illusion perpetrated by the mind in order to distract you from not knowing who you truly are. It does this because lack of identity and self-knowledge is not its responsibility. The mind only exists to help you understand your world, but it cannot reveal to you your true nature. This can only happen once you have removed the veils that obscure your true identity.

In the meantime, the mind's job is to make sense of this lack of identity by identifying instead with what ails the individual, whether it be a financial loss, a failing relationship, or a chronic disease. Once you recognize the signs of victimhood, stop identifying with it, and start seeing through the false-hood of this story. Recognize victimhood for the illusion it is, and unravel why you identify with it.

Identifying with a disease and its symptoms is like being in a storm and taking on the storm as your identity. You only experience the storm; you are not the storm. In the same way, you only experience the illness; it is not who you are. In fact, a storm is a good metaphor to help you visualize your illness for what it is.

Imagine your illness as a swirling mass of dark storm clouds, deafening thunder, blinding lightning, and pelting rain. Feel the fear and anxiety that accompanies such a storm, as it does in a chronic illness. Let the storm batter your body, as does your disease. Feel its wrath, but realize that you are separate from the storm and that it cannot engulf you.

You can get through and overcome the storm, perhaps not completely unscathed but still intact. The same is true for any illness you face, acute or chronic. It can batter you with its onslaught, but it cannot engulf you or break you. You can get through any illness with your body, mind, senses, and spirit intact, just like you can survive any storm. By using this met-aphor, you can unravel your victimization story around your illness and break your identification with it, so it just becomes a passing entity that holds little power over you.

Another common story that people create around their illness is to use it to create a sense of purpose. Not knowing what your life's mission is can allow your disease and symptoms to fill this void and be your life's mission to treat and overcome. The problem is that, at some deep-seated level, you realize that if you ever were to overcome your illness you would lose your sense of purpose. So your life situation plays out in an ongoing struggle between yourself and your symptoms, with a potential treatment or cure always remaining just beyond reach, as a way of sustaining the illness and keeping your life's mission alive.

The way to unravel this story is to realize that your illness and its symptoms are not your life's ultimate mission but are, in fact, keeping you from it. Why do I say this? Note that your illness only affects you; a true life's mission is tied to the greater good. This is why your disease process, although a journey in its own right, can be overcome as you find your life's ultimate mission.

There is one way in which a disease can be your life's ultimate mission, though. That is when you suffer from a rare condition and finding a cure would benefit many others who also suffer from the same condition. You may also be suffering from a common condition, and your life's mission may be to form a support group to help others with the same condition. If these are not true in your case, once you let go of the story of your illness as your life's mission, you are free to let your life's true purpose unfold and to fulfill your ultimate destiny, free of the burden of disease.

Another story often created around illness is feeling that you deserve it. Why would anyone feel that they deserve their disease? Many of us suffer from guilt over something we have done in the past that we may not be very proud of. This often involves having wronged another individual or group of individuals. It may take several forms, such as having ignored your child when he or she really needed your attention but you were too caught up in your own personal issues. You may have emotionally hurt someone who you were once in a relationship with. You may have lied to someone in order to gain an advantage over him or her. You may have physically or sexually abused someone. You may have cheated on your spouse. You may have even murdered someone.

Now by no means am I condoning any of these actions. What I am simply saying is that nobody deserves to be ill or to suffer as a result of their thoughts or actions from the past. We need to realize that we are not perfect and are born to make mistakes, no matter how serious those mistakes are and how deeply they hurt others.

Just as we are not our diseases; we are not our mistakes. Those events that we call mistakes simply took place due to a complex interaction among our circumstances at that time, how we were feeling, our interpretation of the situation, and what we thought we would gain from the thought or act we perpetrated.

Everyone can look back on their lives with regrets; however, the regret we feel is there to teach us important life lessons, not confine us to self-created prisons of shame, guilt, self-loathing, and subsequent chronic stress and disease. Even if you wronged another individual or group of people, you need to see through that event, and all of the negative feelings it brings up inside you, to the lesson it was ultimately meant to teach you. Once you can reframe those negative experiences from your past as valuable life lessons, you no longer need to feel shame or guilt about them and can, thus, let go of the feeling that you deserve to suffer with illness.

Another story that often perpetuates a chronic disease is to use it as a way of getting attention from others. Loneliness has become a pervasive condition in modern society. I believe that its cause is a loss of connection and feeling of oneness with the world, which become replaced by a feeling of separation—from oneself, from other people, from nature, and ultimately, from the universe.

Many people quell their loneliness by using their chronic disease as an attention-getter. I see this all the time in my work as a physician.

At one of the hospitals where I am on call, I regularly treat one patient—I will call her Darlene—who arrives at the emergency room after she has been drinking heavily and called the paramedics. She usually comes in intoxicated, with stable vital signs, no fever, and fairly normal overall diagnostic testing. However, once she is admitted to the ER, she will scream constantly for no particular reason. She is not in pain; she just wants attention. This is why she gets intoxicated and calls the paramedics in the first place.

This is a straightforward example, but many other patients live alone, have multiple medical issues, and end up in the hospital frequently or visit their family physicians more frequently than needed simply to quell their loneliness.

These patients usually have chronic disease and can easily get acutely ill, but the point I am trying to make is that the only human contact they have is when they are at their doctor's office or in the hospital being attended to by healthcare professionals. If they were to fully heal they would lose all human contact, because they would no longer need to be assessed by the healthcare system.

This is a complex problem, with no simple solution, but it all starts with simply recognizing that there is a difference between loneliness and solitude. Loneliness is the feeling that you are an isolated fragment in a hostile universe; solitude is being with oneself in a state of fully embodied presence, wherein, you can start to see your connection, not only to other people but also to nature, the earth, and the entire universe. You can be alone in this state of embodied presence, but because you realize your connection to everything and everyone around you, you are not lonely.

The key to healing the story of loneliness and its connection with chronic disease is to have a direct experience of your connection to everything and everyone. There are many ways to do this. One is to routinely spend time in nature. If you do this often enough, you will experience yourself as part of the natural world and connected to every other living thing.

Another way to do this is to take tiny steps toward connecting with other people. You could start by smiling or saying hello to strangers you encounter daily. As you get more comfortable with this practice, you can progress to initiating small conversations with others. The easiest way to do this is to comment on a positive aspect of that person, such as how well they are dressed, their pretty smile, how well they do their work, their focus and dedication to their craft, or a number of other qualities that can be readily recognized. As you get more comfortable with this, you will naturally find yourself initiating conversations and having more deep and meaningful interactions with others, and soon, your feelings of loneliness will dissipate.

Another story that often drives chronic disease is a feeling of boredom. Often, a patient will have nothing in their life that fills them with drive and passion; they simply drag themselves through every day with a painful lack of enthusiasm. They may not get along with their partner; they may hate their job, they may not have any hobbies or interests and have very little to look forward to in their daily life and near future. So their illness moves in to fill the void created by their boredom.

Why does boredom arise? How can a human being, who is the embodiment of infinite potential, get to a place where nothing interests them?

The answer lies in childhood. As children, we grow up with dreams and aspirations that arise from a sense of wonder at the incredible beauty and possibilities of life. Of course, the child does not understand it this way but simply experiences this as a knowing and certainty that is expressed as pure unbridled joy.

What happens as we grow older is that we lose touch with this sense of wonder and unbridled joy as our responsibilities mount over time. Eventually, life becomes obscured by events and situations that are not sourced directly from life but from the mind's interpretation of reality, which has become filtered through the ego.

This is how our dreams and ambitions become buried and obscured under a heap of daily responsibilities, obligations, material possessions, and false substitutes for what we consider life's greater meaning. As we move away from our childhood dreams, boredom starts to creep into our lives. Eventually, this boredom becomes so prevalent in our daily lives that it needs to be filled with something to occupy its presence, which is often a chronic disease.

The solution to the story of boredom is to rediscover the inner child and to reconnect with our childhood dreams. We can do this by rediscovering the timeless activities that occupied us and filled our days with joy. These may have been playing a specific sport, exploring a nearby creek bed, learning an instrument or just lying in the grass and watching the clouds go by on a bright, sunny day. When you do this, you will start to reconnect with your childhood dreams and rediscover the spark that reignites the source of your joy and sense of wonder.

As you start to rediscover the feelings you experienced as a child, you can start to weave a thread that connects what excited you back then to how you can experience the same feelings now in a more meaningful way.

For example, someone who enjoyed spending time in nature as a child could now start to lead nature walks and retreats for those who are seeking an escape from modern city life. Someone who enjoyed drawing as a child could enroll in art classes and rekindle that childhood passion for art and even begin teaching others how to connect with their artistic creativity. This is how you extinguish your boredom and the void that needed chronic disease to fill it.

Another story often created around one's illness is that of inheritance and thinking that one's family history is a significant factor in predicting the development of chronic disease.

Many of us have parents who suffer from a host of chronic diseases, such as hypertension, diabetes mellitus, coronary artery disease, cerebral vascular disease, chronic obstructive pulmonary disease, peripheral vascular disease, chronic kidney disease, cancer, arthritis, dementia, and other inflammatory diseases.

When we grow up seeing our parents suffer from these conditions, we automatically assume that we are destined to experience the same fate. There are many reasons for this, including hereditary factors, growing up in the same environment with the same diet, and having our habits influenced by our parents. I will address each of these issues, one at a time.

With regard to our genetics, it is no longer true that we are doomed by the genes we inherit. Dr. Bruce Lipton, a renowned cell biologist, has documented this thoroughly in his groundbreaking book, *The Biology of Belief*.

Dr. Lipton took genetically identical stem cells (mother cells that can become any type of cell) and placed them in various culture media to create individual environments for the cells. Depending on the culture medium used, the stem cells became bone, muscle, or fat, which proves that it is the environment not the genetic predisposition of the individual that determines the fate of the cell. This concept is known as epigenetics (from the Greek *epi* meaning "above" genetics), and it has been proven repeatedly that factors in the environment are a greater determinant of the development of disease than genetics alone.

If environment is a significant factor in the expression of our genes, then one may argue that we grow up in the same environment as our parents, so we will experience the same health outcomes. But this is not necessarily true, which I can show from my own example.

I am of South Asian origin and grew up with this kind of diet, which is heavy on red meat, oil-based curries, lots of carbohydrates in the form of various breads, and lots of sweets and desserts. I ate this way for most of my childhood and adolescence until I went away to university, where their dietary influence was not as strong. When I was living at home, I was a chunky child and adolescent, although I did not suffer from many health issues. When I went away to university, I was able to modify my diet over time through healthier choices, eventually increasing my intake of green vegetables, seeds, nuts, berries, and legumes and reducing my intake of red meat, fried foods, carbohydrates, and sweets.

Needless to say, if I had continued on the same dietary trajectory I was on when living at home, I may now be suffering from any number of chronic diseases that I mentioned earlier. If I am able to influence my environment by changing my diet, you can too, and you cannot use the story of family history as an excuse for ill health.

The story of bad genetics and growing up in an unhealthy environment easily falls away in the face of recent scientific evidence to the contrary. If there is any doubt in your mind as to the validity of these claims, then I strongly encourage you to read Bruce Lipton's book, *The Biology of Belief*.

Another story we often tell ourselves when we get chronically ill is that this is how we are meant to age. We may witness this in our parents, in our extended families, and through the media, which is filled with advertisements pushing the newest pharmaceuticals for the next condition we are going to come down with.

When I work in the hospital, I routinely treat patients who are on multiple medications, whose use I frequently question. What has essentially happened is that these patients have been going to their family physicians for years and as new symptoms and complaints arise, new medications get added with no thorough assessment of what medications the patient is on and why they are needed.

I once treated a patient in her mid-eighties with a multitude of symptoms who was on more than thirty medications. I was increasingly convinced that the majority of her symptoms were caused by her polypharmacy and the side effects from the interactions among the medications.

The problem is that most people, as they age, buy into the paradigm perpetrated by our healthcare or disease care system that we will all develop some kind of medical condition eventually. But I challenge this assumption, as there are numerous examples of people who live long and age well without disease.

In his book *Healthy at 100: The Scientifically Proven Secrets of the World's Healthiest and Longest-Lived Peoples*, John Robbins describes the lifestyles and dietary patterns of the long-lived cultures of the Abkhasia of Southern Russia, the Vicalbamba Indians of the Ecuadorian Andes, and the Hunza of Northern Pakistan.

What is common among these cultures is that they consume lower amounts of daily calories than is found in the average western diet, around 1700 to 1800 calories a day, with the majority of their nutrition being plant-based—90 percent for the Abkhasia and 99 percent for the Vicalbamba and Hunza. In addition, these cultures eat low amounts of salt, no sugar or processed food, and have no evidence of obesity and other common chronic diseases in modern society. These cultures also get plenty of exercise through cultivating their land and doing a lot of walking in their beautiful and scenic environments. They also have strong community values, spirituality, and a sense of purpose.

Contrast this with Western culture in which the diet is predominantly meat-based, high in processed foods, with some form of sugar in almost every processed food, and a lot of simple carbohydrates. Furthermore, Western culture favors individuality over community values and materialism over spirituality, all of which contribute to the declining health of members of these cultures as they age.

This should show you that disease as a consequence of aging is not inevitable but associated with an unhealthy lifestyle, as evidenced by the health of elderly members of the cultures I have already mentioned. The story that we have to get sick as we grow older is not borne out by the facts.

As you can see, we create many stories around our chronic diseases, all of which fall apart as we expose the falsehood of these stories and the illusions they perpetuate. As we do so, we find that there is no longer a structure to justify the existence of our disease process, and we may naturally start to experience a resolution of the signs and symptoms associated with the illness.

This is especially true if we have eliminated and reframed our limiting beliefs and burned through our unresolved emotions. Although we may create stories around our chronic illnesses, we should not totally discount our life story. There is meaning and power in our life story, which needs to be harnessed in order to journey toward healing and become whole. This is the topic of the next chapter.

KEY POINTS

- People create many stories about their chronic illnesses, which serve to perpetuate their disease process.
- The common stories people create around disease include being a victim of the disease, the disease creating a sense of purpose, deserving to suffer from the disease, using disease to get attention from others, using disease to alleviate boredom, using disease to perpetuate the false inevitability of genetic inheritance, and justifying disease as a normal part of the aging process.
- These stories can usually be dismantled by delving deeper into them, challenging the assumptions made around them, and exposing them for the illusions that they are.

QUESTIONS TO ASK YOUR CLIENTS

- What are the stories that you have created to perpetuate your chronic illness?
- Is there any validity or truth to your stories?
- Is there any evidence you can find to dismantle the stories you have created around your illness?
- If you were to dismantle the stories you have created around your chronic disease, what would it mean for your overall health?

CHAPTER 13

Narration Part 2 – Seeing Through and Decoding Your Life Story

A t any given point in our lives we all have a life story. This story evolves over time as we accumulate more experiences. People create many archetypal stories based on their life circumstances.

There is the victim story, in which you feel that you are the victim of your parents' upbringing, your childhood experiences, the financial climate in which you were raised, and your lack of opportunities growing up. You feel like everyone is out to get you somehow and you cannot trust anyone.

There is the not deserving story, in which you feel that you do not deserve to be happy, healthy, and living an abundant life, based on guilt or shame over things you may have done in the past.

There is the competition and lack story, in which you feel that you are in competition with everyone else around you for limited resources including consumer goods, financial wealth, love, relationships, and almost anything else you can think of.

There is the power and domination story, in which you feel that you must be in complete control of everyone and everything around you for your life to run smoothly and to take you where you wish to go. If even one thing does not go as expected, you become hopelessly frustrated and feel that all is lost.

These archetypal stories are all rooted in our upbringing and early childhood experiences, as we have already discussed in relation to subconscious blocks and limiting beliefs. Life stories also often revolve around the roles we play in our lives, such as spouse, partner, parent, child, sibling, friend, acquaintance, enemy, employee, manager, or co-worker.

There is nothing wrong with having a story, and we all have them; in fact, nobody can be born into the physical realm without accumulating experiences that culminate in a life story. The problem arises when you start to identify with your life story. Your life story is the accumulation of experiences you have had in the physical realm, but it is not who you are in your essence.

Who you are is far greater than you can ever imagine, and I will try to touch on this in the following chapters. For now, we can say that who you are is pure consciousness, awareness, presence, being, energy, spirit, or a host of other words that we often use to try to unsuccessfully describe the indescribable. The important point is that you are not your life story but the Higher Self that experiences your life story. In essence, you are the observer of the events of your life situation as they unfold over time.

This is a crucial point in the healing journey, because once you have this realization, then you do not have to be defined by your life story and circumstances. Yes, they influence your lower aspects, such as your ego, your mind, and your physical body, but they are not who you truly are. This realization allows you to unleash resources and energies that have been spent upholding and maintaining a false identity and redirect them to go deep within, to the core of your true essence, where the beauty and mystery of life reside.

Once you are able to identify and merge with your essential being, it illuminates the other aspects of yourself and allows you to see them in the context of your true nature or being. In this way, you see your life story as a natural unfolding of your soul's journey in the physical realm, with all its twists and turns, which are meant to wake you up to your true nature.

The other aspect of your life story is the deeper meaning it holds for why you have been birthed into the physical realm. Everything that you have experienced and endured in your life, no matter where it falls on the emotional spectrum, has not occurred randomly or without purpose. Your life events are meant to offer you a greater lesson, whose ultimate purpose is to reveal to you your life's mission.

Every one of you has a reason for being here and a higher mission or purpose, even if you are not aware of this. If you have not discovered your life's mission, it is because you have not scrutinized your life experiences to the degree needed to reveal the greater message that lies behind them. The key to discovering your life's mission is to start to decode your life story by tracing a thread through your life experiences and trying to find the common theme underlying them.

An example of this comes from my own life.

As I mentioned earlier, I was brought up in South Asian Muslim culture, and was clearly a minority in the community where I grew up, with most of my peers being of European origin with Christian-based beliefs. When I went to school and interacted with my peer group, I was exposed to a different culture outside my home. This created a lot of confusion in my early childhood, as I was seen as different and treated as such by my peers, and even by my school teachers. I suffered a crisis of identity, as I felt like I was two different people, depending on the environment I was in. This feeling persisted through my adolescence and early adulthood.

As time passed, I started to feel like I was a bridge between these two worlds and tried to live by integrating the best of both these worlds. The theme of being a bridge has grown as my life story has evolved over time. This has helped unlock my life's greater mission, as I now understand it, which is that I have to be a bridge between modern, conventional medicine and a more holistic, multifaceted, multidimensional approach to health and healing. This does not mean that my life mission will not evolve over time, but this is where my life story has brought me at this point in time.

As we discussed earlier, finding your life's mission by scrutinizing your life's story provides a solid foundation for your intention to heal. It puts any stress in your life into the context of a higher purpose, so that it does not become detrimental to your health but, instead, fuels your life and healing journey.

You can do this by trying to identify a common theme in all of your life experiences and noting which direction they are pointing you in, as I described in my own life story. Use the meditative technique I laid out earlier to enter a state of deep introspection, which will help illuminate the thread that underlies your life story and holds the key to unlocking your life's true mission.

Keep a journal to highlight the common themes that emerge, and try to find the underlying hidden pattern permeating your life experiences. Where have your barriers and challenges been? What can you learn from your triumphs and defeats? What is the underlying lesson that these things have been trying to teach you?

The deeper lessons and underlying thread of your life's experiences may not be readily apparent, but they can be teased out through inner exploration, which may require the services of a coach or mentor. This is crucial work, because it holds the key not only to your health and healing but also to your ultimate happiness, peace, success, and fulfillment.

I started out this chapter discussing the truth of who you are, which underlies your life story. Once you are able to realize this truth, you are then ready for the next step in the healing journey: raising your vibrational frequency.

KEY POINTS

- You are not your life story but the Higher Self that experiences your life story as the experience of your physical self here on the earth.
- You must trace a thread through all of your life experiences in order to find the pattern that will be the key to unlocking the truth of your life's true mission as an expression of your higher purpose.

QUESTIONS TO ASK YOUR CLIENTS

- Who would you be without your life story?
- Can you trace a pattern through all of your past and current life experiences?
- Does this pattern reveal anything to you about your life's greater mission?
- If this pattern does not reveal to you your life's mission, then what are the missing pieces that could lead you to the truth of why you are here?
- How would discovering your life's greater mission transform your experience of life?

CHAPTER 14

Vibration – Increasing Your Personal Energy Vibrational Frequency

Raising your vibration is the next step in your healing journey. Earlier, we discussed that the subatomic particles we are made of only comprise less than a fraction of a percent of the atom, with the majority being empty space. These subatomic particles are essentially packets of energy vibrating at a certain frequency and influencing our experience of life.

If these subatomic particles are vibrating at a low frequency, then we are more likely to feel dense, heavy, anxious, depressed, fatigued, and to become ill. If our subatomic particles are vibrating at a very high frequency, we are more likely to feel light, calm, peaceful, happy, full of energy, and vitality and to remain healthy.

It is very easy in our busy, hectic lives to get bogged down while trying to navigate the challenges of daily life. This is true, even if we have removed our subconscious blocks, rewritten our limiting beliefs, healed our unresolved emotions, and unraveled our disempowering stories.

So why does this happen?

The problem is one of perception. We see ourselves as physical beings made up of bones, organs, and skin, with thoughts, emotions, and desires. We see our job as being to keep our physical bodies healthy in order to be able to pursue our personal desires. Often these desires revolve around wealth, relationships, material possessions, travel, and other pleasures that raise our mood. This is how most people live their lives.

The problem is that most people are seeking certain feelings and validation for their lives through external means. But if you have been at the game of life for some time, you soon learn that no degree of external validation through material seeking and acquiring can bring you these feelings. It cannot even bring them to you transiently.

The reason is that the things most people seek on the physical plane are just faint shadows of what they truly seek. And what do people truly seek? They seek joy, love, and peace, which are essential aspects of who you are at a fundamental level.

We have already discussed how we have the illusion of being physical beings but are really essentially energy beings. Therefore, anything that you do on a physical or material level cannot permanently manifest your true nature of joy, love, and peace. This can only happen through raising your personal vibrational frequency, which can be achieved through several means.

The first involves working with what your physical body ingests and assimilates from the external environment, which is a complicated way of saying eating.

This may seem to contradict what I said earlier about nothing on the physical plane being able to bring you to the high vibrational states of joy, love, and peace. When you see eating as a source of temporary pleasure, such as when you eat desserts and other sugary foods, this is indeed true. Eating these foods can only bring a fleeting sense of happiness not true joy, and this is not the purpose of eating.

The purpose of eating is to take in macro and micro nutrients to feed your body what it needs to stay strong and healthy. Nutrients accomplish this is by being assimilated at the molecular level and supporting optimal cellular function.

Since your cells are made up of molecules, which are in turn made up of atoms, which are in turn made up of subatomic particles, which are just packets of energy vibrating at a certain frequency, your nutrition directly affects your vibrational frequency. This is why people say you are what you eat, which is essentially true, and why it is important to eat foods that will raise your personal vibrational frequency.

So what are these foods?

The way to answer this question is to first discuss which foods will lower your vibration. These are foods that essentially have no nutritional value and are simply ingested for how they taste. These include processed foods, foods with high sugar content, foods high in saturated fat, and unethically raised meat. These have little nutritional value and actually undermine cellular function, thereby, lowering your vibration. They provide absolutely no benefit, yet they are consumed to excess all over the world.

Just look at a typical grocery store, where the majority of food sold is processed and packaged. The food industry thrives on the general population buying what can only be described as "food-like substances," marketed and advertised in such a way that many people are taken in by these poor substitutes for real, natural food. But even though you may get immediate gratification from tasting these foods and satisfying your hunger, the long-term consequences are dire and far outweigh their seeming benefits.

Just look at the health of the average North American, and you will understand what I mean. The decisions to eat these foods are not made from a heart-centered approach but from an egoistic approach, which has no concern for the spirit; it only wants to make you feel instantly better.

So why are our eating habits so bad?

The problem lies with the function of eating itself. We think that eating is something we do to derive pleasure and self-gratification. Just look at the number of restaurants that exist in densely populated areas and their popularity. A whole societal culture revolves around going out to eat. Restaurants are among the most popular places where people go on first dates, get together with friends, and have social gatherings. The problem with this is that we, subconsciously, associate eating at restaurants with enjoyment and pleasure because a lot of our social experiences revolve around these places.

Because of this association, the decisions we make around what food we will eat at these restaurants also is made based on what will be most pleasurable and not on what will be beneficial nutritionally and benefit our personal vibration. In fact, the whole idea of food affecting our vibrational frequency is not a widely known or accepted concept, which is why the consequences of eating are not considered by most people, except when they affect our weight.

However, weight is not the issue. The issue is what food will nourish and support our cells, our immunity, our energy, our spirit, and our personal evolution into fully conscious beings. So how do we support our decisions of what to eat in a more conscious way?

We have already done much of this work by removing our subconscious and emotional blocks and unraveling the stories around our health. A lot of our poor eating habits are based on our emotional traumas and the false stories that form the basis of the decisions we make around our health. I encourage you to go back and re-read the chapters on emotion and narration to refresh your memory, if you need to.

So what foods do truly nourish us at a cellular level, support our immune system, and raise our vibrational frequency? To answer this question, we need to consider two issues. The first issue is the nutritional value of the food we eat; the second issue is the ethical sourcing of our food—the way it was grown or raised.

Let's discuss the first issue in some detail.

I mentioned foods with high nutritional value, but it is not "foods" that we should be ingesting; it is nutrients. By this, I don't mean to imply that we should simply take multivitamins and nothing else; however, it is a scientific fact that some foods are more nutritionally dense than others, and it is a general consensus that the most nutritionally dense foods are plant based.

Leaving aside any food allergies you may have, your nutrition should predominantly be derived from plant sources. Examples of these foods include green leafy vegetables, root vegetables, legumes, fruits (including berries), seeds, nuts, and lentils. Nutritionally poor foods, such as processed foods, gluten-containing grains, dairy products, soy products, genetically modified (GMO) grains and vegetables such as wheat and corn, and simple sugars, should be avoided as much as possible. The book *Super Immunity* by Dr. Joel Fuhrman is an excellent resource on nutrition for optimal health.

At the same time, no discussion of nutrition is complete without a discussion of hydration. It is generally recommended that the average person should drink six to eight 8-ounce glasses of clean, pure water daily.

And now to my second point.

Food needs to be sourced ethically if it is going to raise your vibrational frequency. These days there are many ways in which food is raised unethically. A lot of our produce is genetically modified (GMO), with corn being the prime example. Genetic modification is done to make the crop more resilient to threats from the environment, such as extreme weather, faster to grow, slower to decay, and more plentiful to sell. This is all done in the name of profit, which is the major concern of food corporations.

The problem is that profit trumps all other concerns, including the health consequences of eating GMO foods, which have not been thoroughly researched and whose safety has not yet been determined. Until this is further studied and defined, we have to assume that GMO produce is detrimental to our health and lowers our vibrational frequency and should be avoided at all costs.

Find out where your local grocery store gets its produce and demand that they label all GMO fruits and vegetables. You can also purchase only organic produce, which is sourced naturally (and is by definition non-GMO); although it is more expensive to buy, there is a greater cost to your health and healing to eating GMO produce. If buying organic is too costly, you can always go to your local farmer's market which usually is a venue for local farmers to sell their harvest, most of which is grown naturally and organically.

NOTE: In the United States, look for the distinctive official label on natural foods made from corn, tomatoes, potatoes, and other frequently genetically modified foods that states "Non-GMO"; an increasing number of food companies have signed on to this verification program.

Eating meat raises a whole set of other issues. There are many arguments both for and against eating meat, and I'm not here to advocate for a vegetarian diet. It is, however, generally accepted that most of our protein should come from plant sources. I, therefore, recommend that if you choose to eat meat, it should only comprise approximately 10 percent of your diet and should be used as a condiment and not a main course.

The other problem with meat is that many farm animals are raised with growth hormone to help them grow faster quicker and are also fed antibiotics, which help protect them from infections. Both of these measures are done purely for economic reasons, to protect the investment and secure the profit of industrial farms.

The problem is that we do not know the effects on humans of eating meat raised using this growth hormone. It is clear that giving farm animals antibiotics increases the incidence of antibiotic-resistant bacteria, which can be passed on to humans. In addition, a lot of industrial farm animals are given feed that is genetically modified and raised using chemical pesticides, herbicides, fungicides, and fertilizers. Furthermore, a lot of industrial farm animals are not allowed to roam freely and are treated inhumanely by being kept in confined quarters. In addition, because most of our meat comes from factory farms whose main concern is maximizing their profit, there is no guarantee that their animals don't feel pain or suffer during the slaughtering process.

It is obvious that eating such meat would lower your vibrational frequency; therefore, if you choose to eat meat, I suggest that it should be organically raised. This means that the meat has been raised humanely, with natural feed and without growth hormones or antibiotics. If you are not able to purchase organically raised meat due to limited supply or cost then you should at least settle for grass-fed meat.

Just as eating nutritious foods can raise your vibrational frequency, it follows that using harmful substances can lower your vibrational frequency. These harmful substances include tobacco, alcohol, and illicit drugs, which need to be avoided at all costs.

As a physician, I have treated many patients who are addicted to one or more of these substances. As a pulmonologist, I treat countless patients who suffer from chronic obstructive pulmonary disease, which directly correlates with the amount of tobacco the patient has abused in their life. As a critical care specialist, I have seen many patients who have suffered from alcohol and illicit drug overdoses, as well as the effects of alcohol and narcotic withdrawal.

Often, these patients actually wanted to quit their toxic habit but were unable to because of addiction. Addiction is not just limited to these harmful substances but can also involve food, television, internet, video games, and pornography, to name a few. What I have come to learn is that our approach to treating addiction has been misguided and flawed.

The problem is that addiction is seen as a problem at the level of the physical body, which is viewed as craving the addictive substance or activity. But, as we have already discussed, the physical body is just an illusion as, at the subatomic level, 99.99 percent of who we are is just empty space. Our true nature is that of a vibrational frequency of energy, which is the point of this chapter. Therefore, it follows that our approach to so-called "addiction" should not be focused on treating the physical body but on reinforcing our true vibrational nature.

If avoiding harmful substances and activities could be taught as a means to raise our vibrational frequency, I believe that we would have more success in helping people overcome their addictions. In order to do this, we must give people a direct experience of a higher vibrational frequency and how good it makes them feel and so positively benefits their health. The way to do this is to engage other ways of raising our vibrational frequency;

namely, through manifesting joy and love and expressing gratitude and appreciation. This is the focus of the rest of this chapter.

Imagine that you are seeking joy, and decide to acquire material things that you think will bring you this feeling. To do this, you need to establish a profitable career, which requires a good education. In order to succeed in your educational endeavors, you must work hard. So you start down this whole path to seeking joy by working hard because you feel it will get you to this goal.

Have you ever observed people who are working hard, whether it is for school or work? Most of the time they are under tremendous stress, and this shows in their attitudes and behaviors. There is no inkling of joy in their hard work, even though joy is what they are working toward.

And herein lies the problem. You cannot work to achieve joy through external means, because the things you seek externally to experience joy can easily leave you. You could lose your job due to downsizing, your material possessions could be destroyed in a house flood, and your investments could lose all their value in an economic collapse. Where is your joy now? If it is tethered to external circumstances and rewards, you see how easily it can be destroyed?

So how do you experience joy, if it is not through external means?

It is by realizing that the joy you are seeking is who you truly are. Proof of this can be found in looking at a newborn baby. Except for when babies are hungry, tired, or need to be changed, all they exude is pure joy. Look into a newborn's eyes, and you will have all the proof you need of this fact. The problem arises as the newborn grows into an infant, a child, an adolescent, an adult, and a senior. They accumulate life experiences, some of which are perceived as negative, and this obscures their true nature as joy over time.

The work you have done with removing your subconscious blocks, rewriting your limiting beliefs, healing your unresolved emotions, and unraveling your disempowering stories can remove the layers of density that obscure your true nature as joy. However, what remains to be done is to increase this feeling, which helps raise your vibration.

So how do you manifest the joy that is your true nature and use this to raise your vibration? You do this by expressing the joy that you are in every moment of your life. Life will always present you with situations to express your joy. This could be as simple as appreciating a newly blossoming flower in your garden to experiencing the birth of your newborn baby, and everything in-between.

Start with when you first open your eyes in the morning. Observe the first few rays of sunlight penetrating your curtains through your bedroom window and casting their intricate patterns on everything they illuminate. Watch how these patterns of light evolve as the rays of sunlight increase in intensity with each passing moment.

Notice the items that populate your bedroom, such as your bed, your dresser, your table lamps, and the ceiling fan. Focus on one of them, such as your dresser. Inspect the patterns in the grain of the wood, and bear witness to the intricate beauty of its design. Give thanks to the tree that gave its life so you could have this beautiful piece of furniture which houses your clothes.

As you start to get out of bed and place your feet on your bedroom floor, notice how it feels, the texture of the carpet, or the temperature of the hardwood floor. Feel the sensation fully with every cell in the soles of your feet. As you move to a standing position, notice how your body feels as you support your full weight on your legs. Notice the beauty of movement as you walk toward the bathroom, realizing what a marvel of engineering the human body is. When you turn on the water to wash your face, watch it pour out of the tap and splash onto the sink and send drops of water splattering in all directions. Witness the beauty of this formless substance that we call water, and give thanks for how it nourishes and refreshes you.

When you walk downstairs and enter your kitchen, notice the change in atmosphere as you enter the center of nourishment in your house. Pay attention to whatever food you prepare for breakfast, including its texture, smell, and taste. Feel every morsel of food in your mouth as you chew each bite and as it slips down the back of your throat into your esophagus. Give thanks for the nourishment that this food provides.

As you walk to your garage and open your car door, feel the cold metal of the door handle. As you open the door and enter your car, notice the comfort you feel in this familiar setting, which you experience every work day. Feel the engine come to life as you turn your ignition key, its raw power as you push down on the accelerator.

As you pull out of your driveway, feel the road under your wheels with every change in its contours. Feel the sun shine on your face and arms through your car windows, or notice the rain obscure your windshield before your wipers clear away the numerous droplets. As you drive to work, pay close attention to the world around you—the houses, buildings, trees, other cars, and people. Try to notice things that you may not have paid attention to in the past, and take in the sublime beauty of the world around you.

As you get to work and go about your day, give the rest of your day the same attention to detail that you did from the time you woke up to the time you arrived at your workplace, and carry this practice onward in every moment of your life.

What is the purpose of this exercise and how does it relate to joy? The purpose of this exercise is to experience the stark beauty in every moment of your life, and let these moments ignite the joy that lies within you. This is how you realize yourself as pure joy.

A second way to raise your personal vibration is to manifest the love that you are. Let's delve into this more deeply.

Most people's experience of love has to do with seeking other people's love. This is usually done through engaging in romantic relationships, which are the most complex aspects of anyone's life. When you first meet someone you are attracted to, you are in a state of ecstasy and nothing can bring you down. Colors look brighter, food tastes better, you are more productive at work, and you are full of energy and feel unstoppable. These feelings usually persist as you enter into a relationship, and you are on top of the world. As time passes, the initial passion eventually wears off and then reality sets in. You start to notice your partner's idiosyncrasies, and things that you initially ignored start to bother you. His snoring may annoy you; you may get irritated with his bathroom habits; you have to clean up after him in the kitchen; you may notice that his work never ends, even when he is home, and any number of other issues that always emerge over time.

The initial love you felt when you first met him does not hold the same intensity. But is this the other person's fault? Is this the nature of relationships? Are all relationships always destined to turn sour? The answer to all these questions is no.

The problem is that you are seeking something through external means that cannot be found outside of yourself, namely love. Love is not found through relationships, external validation or through other people's approval. Love is only found within yourself as your essential nature, and manifests through expressing it in the world. If you do not realize and practice this, your relationships will always disappoint you, because you will use them to seek what they cannot give you. Therefore, the purpose of relationships is to provide a vehicle to express the love that you are, not to seek it by entering them.

This is the reason why many relationships and marriages fail. Imagine how your relationships could transform if you realized this and lived according to the principle of love being your true nature? Imagine the feelings of ecstasy, passion, and fulfillment persisting throughout the duration of any relationship you engage in, instead of fizzling out over time. Imagine seeing the world through the eyes of love. Imagine if the majority of the world's population understood this principle and lived according to it. Our world would transform from one of turmoil, conflict, and misery to one of peace, serenity, and joy.

What would be the effect on your health if you lived from a place of pure love? This would naturally raise your vibrational frequency and make you less susceptible to acute illness and chronic disease and, thus, improve your overall health.

So how do you manifest the love that you are? You do this by showering everyone and everything around you with compassion and kindness, not just the one who is your life partner. There is no shortage of opportunities to express compassion and kindness in our world, which seems to be so full of pain and suffering. From holding the door open for strangers to volunteering at a food bank, there are many ways to show your compassion and kindness to those who need it. All you have to do is open your eyes and look around you to find these opportunities.

Some examples of such opportunities are:
- Reading books to children at your local library
- Spending time with a lonely senior at a nursing home
- Reaching out to family members with whom you have not communicated in a long time
- Listening deeply to a friend or colleague who is going through a difficult time in his or her life
- Helping a neighbor mow his lawn or shovel snow off his driveway
- Helping to feed the needy at your local food bank

- Becoming a Big Brother or Big Sister to a lonely child
- Helping to care for a chronically ill grandparent
- Becoming a foster parent
- Volunteering at your local animal shelter
- Hosting a neighborhood barbecue to promote a sense of community
- Showing your partner compassion, even when they are upset with you
- Buying your co-workers coffee
- Giving your partner a gift without a special occasion
- Saying some kind words to someone who is in emotional pain from a major loss

These are just a few of the countless ways you can express the love that you are. You will find that as you walk this path of expressing your unconditional love, it will become your natural state once again, as it was always meant to be. This will raise your vibrational frequency, and you will reap the health benefits that follow.

A third way to raise your personal vibration is through the practice of gratitude. Gratitude is simply being thankful for everything and anything you have. It does not matter what your situation is or how much lack you perceive in your life, there is always someone who has less than you do. Therefore it is important to be grateful for what you do have, no matter how little it might be.

Gratitude attunes you to the source of all that is, whether you want to call that source God, Nature, or the Universe. Once you have attuned to that source, abundance can flow naturally to you and further enrich your life. Furthermore, being attuned to the highest source will naturally raise your vibrational frequency.

One way to do this is to start a daily practice in which you give gratitude for at least one thing in your life. For example, some of the things you may be grateful for are:

- The oxygen you breathe
- The nutritious food you eat daily
- The roof over your head
- Having a wonderful life partner

- Your beautiful children, or nieces and nephews if you have none of your own
- Having a means of earning a decent living
- Having great friends and family
- The wonder of technology and how it has revolutionized how you live your life
- Your free time, when you are able to pursue your personal interests at leisure.
- Your eyesight to witness the beauty in the world
- Your hearing ability to be able to listen to others
- The gift of language and communication
- Your ability to walk and the complexity of movement that your body can experience
- Your ability to think and use your mind to solve complex daily problems
- The gift of humor and the ability to laugh
- The gift of sadness and the ability to work through grief over a loss
- Your place in nature, with the ability to become aware of your higher consciousness
- The gift of choice in all aspects of your life
- Being embodied in human form in order to experience life on Earth
- The gift of intuition and how it can guide you in your daily life

And these are just some aspects of your life that you can be grateful for. As you start to show daily gratitude for all that you have and experience, you open a conduit to the Source of all that is. This allows more abundance to flow into your life and illuminate every aspect of your being. It will raise your vibrational frequency and catapult you into higher levels of health and well-being.

What follows the high vibration of gratitude is the high vibration of appreciation. Appreciation occurs when your ongoing practice of daily gratitude coalesces into a constant state of genuine gratefulness and wonder, as you recognize the glorious miracle that life is. Appreciation should extend to all aspects of your life, including the aspects that may appear challenging. For example, if you are in a romantic relationship and are experiencing some conflict with your partner, you should appreciate this. This turbulence in your relationship is there to help you understand your partner better, for you to grow in your relationship, and to learn more about yourself.

If you are in the midst of financial struggle you should appreciate this, because this experience is meant to help you learn how to effectively manage your money and to manifest your abundance in more creative and innovative ways. This struggle may eventually lead you to new frontiers that you may have never considered, such as relocating to a new country, starting a new business venture right where you are, or leaving your job to seek more freedom to do the things you love to do. These experiences in turn will push you beyond your comfort zone and contribute to your growth. By appreciating everything in your life, you will shift your vibrational frequency in a way that will help you navigate any challenges or obstacles in your life with greater grace and ease.

Just imagine how your physiology could change as you embody appreciation, and it becomes your natural state of being. If you were to combine the embodiment of joy, love, gratitude, and appreciation the possibilities for your health would be limitless.

The key to achieving these levels of unbelievable health is to start embodying one of these aspects of yourself through the practices I have already discussed and to gradually embody all four of these aspects over time. As you do this, you will start to enter and experience the state of flow, which is the subject of the next chapter.

KEY POINTS

- At the fundamental level, our true nature is that of a vibrational frequency of energy.
- Our vibrational frequency is the source of our experience of our life.
- One way we can raise our vibrational frequency is through the food we choose to eat.
- Avoiding harmful substances will also raise our vibrational frequency, but this often requires a direct experience of a high vibrational frequency.

- We can also raise our vibrational frequency by expressing joy, love, gratitude, and appreciation in our daily lives.

QUESTIONS TO ASK YOUR CLIENTS

- What is the fundamental nature of who you truly are?
- Is your current nutrition supporting your highest vibrational frequency?
- If not, then what changes could you make in your nutritional choices to increase your vibrational frequency?
- Are there any addictive substances or activities you are engaged in that are lowering your vibrational frequency?
- How can you truly break free of these addictions?
- How can you experience joy in every moment of your life?
- What can you do to express the love that you are?
- What are you grateful for in this very moment?
- Can you find something to be grateful for every day of your life?
- What are some of the things that you appreciate in your life?
- Are you able to appreciate your personal challenges by allowing them to reveal their deeper purpose in your life?
- How would your experience of life transform if you were to find a way to appreciate your life's personal challenges?

CHAPTER 15

MOTION –
ENTERING THE FLOW

Flow, by definition, is the state of complete synchronicity of an organism or individual, both within itself and with its external environment. Let's look at this more closely from the perspective of the individual.

Your natural state is that of flow. All of our physiological processes depend on flow, from the most basic processes, such as cellular communication, to the more complex processes, such as circulation and breathing.

As we discussed earlier, the most basic unit of matter is the atom. Its subatomic particles are simply packets of energy that are in a constant state of flow, with fluctuating vibrational frequencies.

If you examine the most basic unit of life, the cell, it is made up of cytoplasm and intracellular organelles. The cytoplasm is in a constant state of flow, carrying nutrients, electrolytes, and proteins encoded by the DNA. Cells communicate with each other through chemical signals that bind to proteins on the cell surface. This turns on a signaling cascade that ultimately leads to the cell's response. This process occurs through a constant state of flow. Multicellular organisms such as ourselves rely on flow in order to survive. The flow of oxygen travels from the air into the upper airway into the lower respiratory passages and to the basic units of the lung, the alveoli. Here, the oxygen is absorbed across the alveolar and capillary endothelia into the bloodstream, where it attaches to the hemoglobin portion of the red blood cells.

The flow of blood carries oxygen to all the various organs and cells of the body through an intricate network of blood vessels called capillaries. This same network of blood vessels carries carbon dioxide from the cells to the lungs to be expired into the air. This flow of blood is continuously driven by the pumping of your heart. It is this same flow of blood that carries the waste products of cellular metabolism to be excreted by the kidneys.

Numerous biofeedback loops in the human body operate in a state of flow. For example, the hormone cortisol, produced by the adrenal glands, is stimulated by the hormone adrenocorticotropin, which is produced by the anterior pituitary, which is, in turn, stimulated by corticotropin releasing hormone, produced by the hypothalamus. If increased production of cortisol is needed in times of heightened metabolism, more corticotropin releasing hormone is produced, which stimulates the production of more adrenocorticotropin, which in turn stimulates more cortisol production, all in a biofeedback loop. This is known as the HPA axis and is just one of the many biofeedback loops in the human body that depend on a state of flow.

Any disruption in flow can lead to dysfunction and disease. For example, airflow obstruction in the airways of the lung is what characterizes asthma or chronic obstructive pulmonary disease, which are both pathologic conditions of the airways. Any impediment to blood flow in your blood vessels is what leads to ischemia, which is tissue damage from lack of oxygenation. Any disruption in intracellular communication can also lead to dysfunction of the tissues and organs involved and hence a disease state. As you can see, flow is vital to maintain the integrity of function of the human body, or of any organism for that matter.

If you examine all of nature, it exists in a constant state of flow. Take, for example, the water cycle. The heat of the sun causes water from streams, rivers, lakes, and oceans to evaporate. The evaporated water will eventually rise and form clouds. At a certain level of humidity in the atmosphere, the clouds will produce rain, which fall on mountains, valleys, forests, and vast plains. This water will eventually feed streams, which feed rivers, which feed lakes and larger bodies of water, namely seas and oceans, and the cycle starts again.

Plants and trees also exist in a cycle. Trees start to grow leaves in the spring, which eventually become abundant and bring the tree to life in the late spring and early summer. It is the leaves that allow the plants and trees to carry out the complex process of photosynthesis, which converts light energy into chemical energy for plants and trees to survive and thrive. In the fall, the leaves start to change color and eventually fall off the branches and become decaying vegetative matter. It is this vegetative matter that provides nutrients to the roots of trees, which allows the cycle to start again the following spring.

Daily human life also needs to remain in a state of flow in order to function effectively. Clogs in your plumbing pipes can cause water to back up, resulting in a flood in your home. Too high a resistance in an electric circuit, such as running too many appliances at the same time, can cause a short circuit, triggering the circuit breakers, and completely shutting down the electric circuit. If there is a mechanical problem on an assembly line of a manufacturing plant, it can delay production for hours and possibly longer. If an accident on a major highway blocks one or more lanes, traffic can become backed up for miles. If money does not circulate freely in our economy, such as when it is being squandered by the few who are in power and wealthy, the economy stagnates, since the majority will not have the finances to buy goods and services. Eventually interest rates will have to drop to re-stimulate financial growth. Even the world beyond our planet is in a constant state of flow as the planets in our solar system all orbit the sun in an organized fashion and never fall out of orbit or threaten to cross paths with one another.

If all aspects of life in the universe thrive in a state of flow then it only makes sense that you, as a human being on this planet, can only also thrive in a state of flow. As I have already discussed, all of our bodily processes, from the subatomic level to the organ system level, depend on flow in order to maintain a healthy state. Flow is our natural state, but modern life easily takes us out of this state with all of its demands, pressures, and distractions.

So how do you maintain flow in every aspect of your being? You do this by being in the moment. What do I mean by being in the moment? The moment is where the past, present, and future coalesce into the now. The moment is where all separation ends between one human being and another. The moment is where you are one with nature and the entire universe. The moment is where there is complete synchronicity in all aspects of your life. The moment is where you transcend time. When you transcend time, you transcend cause and effect, which is the usual paradigm of disease manifestation.

The paradox of disease is that it develops over time but can only be healed by being in the moment, that place where you are in a constant state of flow. Lamenting over the past diminishes the energy of flow. Worrying about the future diminishes the energy of flow. Seeing yourself as separate from all others and from nature diminishes the energy of flow. Therefore, being in the moment is the key to being in the flow and healing chronic disease, as disease is a state of stagnation that is contrary to flow.

Very few people experience living at a deeper level. That's because most people are too busy skimming the surface of life, caught up in distractions, such as work issues, daily chores, paying the bills, shuttling kids between activities, home renovations, car maintenance, keeping their significant other happy, meal planning, finding time to exercise, getting to doctors' appointments, and finding time to get enough sleep. Don't get me wrong. I am not denying the importance of these daily activities. What I am saying is that these activities occupy so much of our time that most of us never experience life at a deeper level.

A metaphor to illustrate this more effectively is the ocean. If you think of the surface of the ocean, it is like the lives that most of us lead. When the ocean is calm, you seem to be in the flow, riding the gentle waves, and letting them take you where they may. This is analogous to the times in your life when all is going well.

However, it is not long before the sky becomes cloudy and dark, thunder rumbles, and you see flashes of lightning in the distance. The ocean, which was once calm, starts to become choppier, and the waves become stronger and more unpredictable as it starts to rain. Soon you are being tossed, turned, and thrown from one place to another in a chaotic pattern with no sense of flow.

This is analogous to those times in your life when things fall apart and nothing seems to be working. You have relationship issues, problems at work, ill health, and financial limitations, to name a few of the things that can go wrong in daily life. But if you were to dive down below the surface of the ocean, you would find a place of serenity and peace similar to what you experienced on the ocean's surface before the storm hit.

The surface of the ocean can change in an instant, whereas beneath the waves, the ocean remains calm and serene, regardless of what is happening on the surface. This constant flow is maintained, no matter how deep you dive into the ocean. You can experience the same flow in your daily life by diving into the depths of your life and experiencing being in the moment in the core of your being.

So how do you embody the moment at the deeper level needed to be constantly in the flow? By focusing on both your inner milieu and your outer circumstances. To do this successfully, what is required is not meditation but attention. Most of us are only focused on our outer circumstances, but to experience flow you must explore the depths of your inner world in the moment.

What populates your inner world is mainly thoughts and emotions. So to plunge into the depths of life, you must focus on your thoughts and emotions as they arise from moment to moment, regardless of what they are. The goal of this exercise is not to change your thoughts and emotions, but to bring them to consciousness by illuminating them.

Cultivating focused attention is much easier than it seems. You can start by being aware of what you are feeling in the moment. It does not matter if you are feeling elated or desolate. The key is to become aware of what you are feeling. Becoming aware of your feelings puts them into perspective and allows you to experience them in the context of the depths of your inner being, which becomes further illuminated as you plunge deeper.

Start by becoming aware of every thought that passes through your mind and watching for the next thought that enters your consciousness. This could be the conversation you had with your boss the previous day, what you should cook for dinner tonight, the next chore or errand you have to complete, or what you are doing right now. Just watch your mind for the next thought that enters it, no matter what it is and observe it fully without judging it.

As you cultivate this mindfulness practice, you will find yourself excavating the depths of an inner world you scarcely knew existed. You will be able to see that your thoughts and emotions are entities that you experience, but that they are not who you are in your true essence, which will be revealed to you as something that transcends your thoughts, emotions and your physical form. As this revelation manifests in your consciousness, so will your true nature as a rhythm of constant flow that is naturally healing.

As you progress in this practice of focused attention on your inner world and realize yourself as a rhythm of constant flow, you will start to see your outer world align in your favor. You get a random phone call from someone who can help you with a problem you are having, a check arrives in the mail with the right amount of money you need to pay a bill, a book falls off the shelf in front of you at the bookstore that addresses issues in your life that you are currently struggling with, to name just a few of the synchronicities that can grace you in the flow. In the rhythm of constant flow, your life takes on a pattern that guides you in your daily routines toward your ultimate destiny, whatever that may be and, ultimately, heals you.

The next level of practice to get into the flow involves your body and its physiologic functions. Getting your physiology into the flow is ultimately how you will maintain your health and prevent chronic disease, because great health is ultimately about being in the flow.

One way to get your body into the flow is to focus on your breath. Breath is the flow of oxygen-rich air from the environment into your lungs. By focusing on your breath, you are experiencing the flow in its most basic form. You don't need to breathe deeply or in any special way; just focus on your breath.

As you inhale, feel the flow of air moving from your immediate environment past your lips, into your mouth, through your pharynx, your larynx, through your trachea, into your proximal airways, into your distal airways, into the tiny air sacs called alveoli where the oxygen is absorbed into your bloodstream through the walls of tiny blood vessels called capillaries. Experience the same flow with exhalation, as the air leaves your lungs and eventually exits your mouth through the same trajectory in the opposite direction.

This is the most basic cycle of life you can experience. Focusing and mindfully experiencing your breath is a practice that you can do anytime and requires only the effort of your attention. The more you bring your attention back to your breath, the more you directly experience the flow manifest in physical form.

Another way of experiencing flow is to visualize the circulation in your body. Your circulation is the ultimate manifestation of flow. It transports oxygen from your lungs and nutrients from your intestines to all the organs, tissues, and cells of your body, then carries away the waste products of metabolism from your cells to your lungs and kidneys. It is integral to your health.

You cannot directly feel your circulation in the way you can feel your breath flowing into and out of your lungs, so you must experience the flow of your blood through visualization. The way to do this is to first feel the pulse, somewhere in your body. The easiest place to do this is in your wrist on your thumb side, which is where your radial pulse is located.

Once you can feel your pulse, focus on each beat of your pulse. Feel the blood coursing through your vessels, and realize that each rush of blood through your arteries begins with the beating of your heart, the origin of your circulation. Realize that these arteries reach all of your organs and tissues through smaller blood vessels called capillaries, with veins returning the blood to your heart. In total, your blood vessels are 100,000 kilometers long, a miracle in itself. Picture the blood flowing smoothly and effortlessly through your vessels with no impediment or obstacle. Just as your breath is integral to life, as it helps oxygenate your blood, your circulation is also integral to life, as it carries the oxygen to all the cells of your body. Therefore flow is vital to your optimal health.

Another manifestation of flow in the body is the cerebrospinal fluid, or CSF, a clear, watery fluid that is produced from arterial blood by structures in the brain called choroid plexuses in the lateral and fourth ventricles. The CSF is produced and circulates through the ventricles of the brain and the subarachnoid space of the meninges, the three membranes that cover and protect the brain and spinal cord. Absorption of CSF into the bloodstream primarily takes place in the superior sagittal sinus through granulations called arachnoid villi and along the nerve roots of the spinal column.

The CSF has several functions, including buffering the brain to prevent injury, excretion of waste products into the bloodstream, as a medium to transport hormones and nutrients, and to support the central nervous system.

Again, here is an example of how flow is vital to health, in this case, the health of the brain and the whole body. To experience this flow, visualize the CSF as it is produced and circulates to the various parts of your brain and spinal cord. Focus on the upper part of your head, on your brain, and put all of your attention there. You may start feeling a tingling sensation in your scalp as you become aware of this flow of CSF and how important it is to brain health. Feel the CSF as it flows to all parts of your brain and protects and nourishes this vital organ and travels down the spinal column to your sacrum, protecting your spinal cord and entire central nervous system.

Focus and attention on your breath, your blood circulation, your lymphatic circulation, your CSF circulation, and other examples of flow in your body will not only enhance and maintain these aspects of flow but keep you in the flow as a human being on this planet.

The next level of manifesting flow is through movement. Movement is how your body maneuvers itself through this physical world we live in. Movement is something many people have lost touch with in our vehicle-bound, internet-addicted, desk job lives. Movement was once an integral part of life among our ancestors who were nomads and followed herds of animals across vast plains and forests in order to stay close to a key source of food. Our ancestors also had to be on the move to meet other needs of basic living, including foraging for wild edibles, gathering shelter building materials, collecting firewood, and being on the lookout for danger from enemy tribes.

As we transitioned from a hunter-gatherer society to an agricultural society, there was less of a need to be on the move as food could be grown and livestock could be raised for meat. Each subsequent era in human history, namely the industrial age, the technological age, and the information age has resulted in a decrease in the need for movement and hence a cessation of this aspect of flow. This is contrary to our nature as physical beings, because our bodies are designed for movement, and when they are not utilized to their fullest extent, stagnation results and all the ill health effects that follow.

I'm not suggesting that we revert to being hunter-gatherers but that we embrace the sacred practice of bodily movement in our daily lives. This could take the form of something as simple as walking along a nature trail to more complex practices such as yoga, tai chi, or other martial arts. It could also be through fitness training or team sports. The important thing is to get up off your couch or chair and move.

Movement should be engaged in as regularly as possible—several times a day, if possible—and is a simple practice to cultivate. Examples of integrating movement into your daily life include parking far from the grocery store so you have to walk more, using the stairs at work instead of the elevator, using your work lunch break and other breaks to do quick power walks, getting a standing workstation at your job, walking around your house or backyard in the evening instead of sitting in front of the television, to name just a few ideas.

Once movement is integrated into your daily life, you may want to engage in a more formal movement practice such as simple stretching, brisk walking, hiking, yoga, tai chi, martial arts, or any number of sports that you can enjoy. The key to sustaining a regular practice of movement is to make it fun and social so it is enjoyable and not something that you have to mentally struggle to do. In this regard, each person's movement practice will be uniquely suited to their interests and needs.

Movement is an external manifestation of flow that is expressed through your body and serves to keep you in the universal flow, which ultimately is healing and health promoting. When we discuss movement, we also have to address the issue of adequate rest for the body, which is between ten and twelve hours of sleep for children and seven to nine hours of sleep for adults. This is essential to maintain flow through movement during the day.

The next level of manifesting flow is in your external environment. This refers to how you move through your daily routines at home and at work. Unfortunately, modern human society has become so dysfunctional and chaotic that it is not easy to experience the state of flow in our daily lives in this world. This is not to say that it is not possible to find pockets of experience when you are in the flow, such as when you are able to navigate a traffic jam in the morning to get to work on time, when you are able to land a major contract at work with very little effort, or you are in the zone in your weekly pickup basketball game and score multiple baskets to secure your team's victory.

However, being in a state of continuous flow is not the norm in most people's daily lives, nor in our society at large, which always seems to be in a state of turmoil and chaos. This is why attention and focus is needed to manifest the rhythm of constant flow in your daily external environment.

But what should you be focusing on to experience this state of flow?

The key to knowing this is to go back to a situation when you were "in the zone," which is akin to being in the flow. We all can recall such experiences from our past, even though they may be few and far between. However, it is not a multitude of such occurrences that you need to remember but just the one that resonates with you so strongly that you remember it as if it has just happened yesterday.

I want you to close your eyes and scrutinize every detail of this experience in your mind's eye. Remember how you felt, what you were thinking, how you moved, how you engaged with others involved, and how the event in question transpired.

What you will likely recall is that you navigated through the situation effortlessly without even having to think. You were in complete synchronicity with the situation that presented itself. Was this due to your knowledge, skills, and effort? Certainly, these factors are necessary ingredients to achieve goals, but they do not guarantee success. Success is achieved when you are in the flow and in the zone, and this can only be achieved when you are willing to let go of the need for any specific outcome and let the situation live you.

Let me repeat that, because it is a crucial distinction to understanding how to achieve the state of flow in the external environment. You cannot live the situation; you must let the situation live you.

What does this mean? It means that you are in such synchronicity with what you are doing and your surroundings that all separation vanishes and you are one with everyone and everything involved. Your environment simply becomes an extension of who you are and takes on a life of its own, which guides your thoughts and actions in the moment. This is how the situation lives you, and you enter the flow. This is a paradigm shift in how to live moment by moment in our daily lives, and in stark contrast to the way most of us live.

Most people see their daily routines as a struggle against others and time and toil through their day. Living this way will only serve to augment your stress level and keep you chronically ill. This new way of living—as though everyone and everything is an extension of yourself—is meant to help you navigate through your daily life. The energy of everyone and everything around you will feed your energy and conspire to keep you in the flow, and this is when you experience being in the zone.

The way to embody this experience is to do a simple exercise. When you have some free time in the day, preferably in the morning before your routine starts, sit in a quiet place and look around you and everything in your immediate vicinity. Picture all the things in your environment as an extension of your being, including the air around you. Realize that the separation you perceive is simply an illusion and that you are truly one with everyone and everything, including the people and things that you cannot perceive with your five senses. Let this realization sink into your consciousness, so that it permeates your being right to the core.

Do this exercise for at least five minutes on a daily basis, preferably in the morning and at night. As you go about your daily routine, realize this oneness with everyone you encounter, from the other drivers on your route to work to your co-workers and the people who you communicate with by phone and by email. Realize your oneness with the earth, the sky, and everything in-between that you can perceive with your five senses. This way, you will be able to embody the rhythm of flow in your daily routine.

In addition to what I have just discussed, the other place where you can experience the rhythm of constant flow is in nature. Nature that is unperturbed by human activity is always in total harmony. The plants, trees, insects, birds, animals, rivers, lakes, valleys, and mountains all depend on and support one another and embody the state of flow.

By spending more time in nature you can anchor this state of flow into your being and progress on your healing journey. There is no special method or process to engage in the flow of nature. All that is needed is a free spirit, an open mind, and an area of unperturbed wilderness, or something close to it. Enter this sanctuary of nature on a regular basis, preferably for at least thirty minutes a day or for as much time as you can devote in the beginning.

As you enter nature's sanctuary, use all five of your senses to hone your awareness to your natural surroundings. Use your sight to take in the trees, plants, birds, wildlife, clouds, and weather formations. Pay attention to the details you see, including colors, textures, patterns, and the randomness of nature. Notice the birds that frequent this patch of nature, where they nest, the extent of their territory, what they feed on, and how they react to you. Over time, you will learn not to instigate alarm calls from the birds you encounter by increasing your zone of awareness.

Listen to the sounds of nature. Hear the wind rustling through the leaves, and listen to the birds and their various calls, including how they react to you. Hear the rushing water, as the river runs its course through the landscape. Try to distinguish the different animals from the sounds they make and what each sound means. Most important of all, listen closely to those moments of silence that are experiences in nature, and notice the depth of that silence and how it speaks volumes that can reveal to you nature's secrets.

Use your sense of smell to take in all of nature's scents, from the fragrance of flowers to the stench of a dead animal. All of it is profound and can be a key practice to help you connect to nature.

Use your sense of touch to physically feel the plants, trees, flowers, and the earth itself. Feel the texture of everything you touch and what information nature conveys to you through this sense. It is unlikely that a bird will land on your hand or that you will get close enough to a wild animal to touch it; however, if you are lucky enough to have this experience, bask in the wondrous glow of this level of connection to nature.

As you navigate your small part of nature, use all of your senses to analyze, interpret, and immerse yourself in your surroundings. Do not simply be a traveler briefly passing through nature, but become one with the natural world, which is the source of our origin. As you start to experience oneness with the natural world, you will enter the flow in which nature resides and functions at all times, if left unperturbed.

Imagine how your life would change if you were able to embody external flow in the way I have described. Imagine how this would transform your personal relationships with your family, friends, and peers, which would become more focused on mutual cooperation instead of adversarial. Imagine how this would transform your home life, your work environment, and your leisure time, which would become more enjoyable and less stressful.

Imagine how embodying external flow would change interactions and dealings at the highest levels of society in politics, business, and philanthropy, which would become more about what we can give, not what we can get. Imagine how this would change the relationships between nations and war and conflict, which would become more about what is right and not just about who is right. Imagine how embodying external flow would change athletic competition, which would become about an interplay of energy between opponents rather than about destroying your adversary. Competition would continue as before, but victory would be determined by who is more in the flow. Imagine how life on our planet could potentially be transformed through the practice of flow at all levels of being, individually, collectively, and globally.

As you embody the flow at all levels of your being, your inner world of your thoughts and emotions, your cellular and higher physiology, your body's movements through the world and your external societal and natural environment, this flow will become your natural state and conspire to keep you in a complete state of health and well-being. This will also transform your relationship to people around you, your immediate environment, and the world at large in a positive way. The more people who embody the flow in this way, the more widespread will be the positive impact and the overall benefit for humanity as a whole.

KEY POINTS

- Flow is the natural state of the entire universe.
- Flow in your life is manifested at multiple levels, including your inner world of thoughts and emotions, your physiology, your body's movements, and how you navigate your external reality in your daily life.
- There are several practices that you can engage in to embody flow at the various levels of your being.
- The manifestation of flow in your external reality is commonly known as the experience of being in the zone.
- If more people were to embody the flow at all levels of their being, life on our planet would be transformed, to the benefit of all of humanity.

QUESTIONS TO ASK YOUR CLIENTS

- Do you remember a time when you were completely in the flow?
- Do you remember what you were thinking, how you felt, and what you were focusing on in the moment that you were in the flow?
- Can you see that flow is the natural state of your body's physiology and is essential for your optimal health?
- What are some of the ways in which you could embody flow in your life?
- How would your life transform if you were to see everyone and everything around you as simply an extension of yourself?
- How would you integrate these practices to enter the flow into your daily life?
- How can you consistently get into and stay in the zone?
- How would being in the flow transform your relationships with those closest to you, your immediate environment, and the world at large?
- How would our world transform if more and more people were consistently in the flow?

CHAPTER 16

Realization – Embracing the Unknown

The step of realization occurs naturally after embodying the state of flow, and it relates to your relationship to the unknown. We visited this step earlier in this process after setting our intention to heal. However, at that stage, you were still in a state of fear of the unknown, as you were still conditioned by your subconscious limiting beliefs, unresolved emotions, identification with false narratives, low vibrational frequency, and not being in the flow. From that place, the unknown is a dark and scary void where few dare to tread. This resistance to the unknown ties up a lot of energy and can accelerate the progression of chronic disease in many ways.

First, fear causes resistance, which causes stress, and stress has been implicated as a major factor in promoting and perpetuating chronic disease. Second, the energy used in resisting the unknown takes energy away from the healing of any ailment you may be suffering from. Third, when you are dealing with illness, you are essentially entering into the unknown, and you need to be able to navigate this uncertain territory in order to effectively engage your illness.

When there is lack of insight and the truth is obscured, this can lead to fear and resistance to the unknown, but once you have excavated the depths of your inner world, as we have been doing up till now, fear starts to drop away. As the fear drops away, so does the resistance to the unknown and you naturally embrace the unknown without any thought or care for what might be awaiting you on the other side of uncertainty. In fact, it is at the edge of uncertainty that life is fully experienced and true healing can occur.

The true nature of life is uncertainty. Although we like to believe that we know where we are headed and what to expect in the seconds, minutes, hours, and days ahead, the truth is that the plans we make for our lives are only meant to distract our minds from the true nature of reality.

Our minds need to be distracted from reality because reality is a concept that is too vast for the mind to comprehend, and that becomes the source of its fear. The truth is that the mind is too limited to wrap its understanding around the nature of existence. It's true strength lies in its ability to navigate the practical aspects of our daily lives in the physical plane.

In order to embrace the unknown, we need to find that place deep within ourselves that is akin to the unknown. This is a part of ourselves that few people ever get to know and truly experience. It is the void from which we emerged, the same void from which the universe was created, through the Big Bang. No scientist truly understands what the Big Bang was and how it led to the creation of the universe. However, I do not believe that our understanding of this phenomenon lies in scientific scrutiny but lies in entering the void where all logic and rationale fall away.

This void runs as deep in our own being as the vastness of the universe, wherein lies both the beauty and mystery of life and the nature of existence. Because the void or the unknown is the source of all of creation, negation of this aspect of ourselves solidifies the illusion that we are our bodies, our thoughts, and our emotions. The truth is that these are only aspects of who we are; they are not our true nature. By believing in the illusion of their reality, we reinforce the negation of the truth of who we truly are. The truth of who we are is indescribable and incomprehensible by the mind, which is why few people ever experience the depths of their true nature.

If we truly understood our true nature and the vastness of our magnificence, the issues that occur in our daily physical lives would reveal themselves to be tiny drops of water that are easily swallowed up by the vast ocean of reality. These issues include our illnesses, which affect the illusory aspects of ourselves, our bodies, our minds, and our feelings.

This may seem callous and insensitive to those who are reading these words, but this is only because we have grown up believing in the falsehood of who we think we are and ignoring the depths of our true reality. This is not our fault, as we have been raised in a world that believes in the illusion and is ignorant of the true nature of its existence. If we can embrace the mystery of who we are, which eludes our rational understanding, we can source our lives from this infinite realm and truly transcend our illnesses.

If we do not embrace the mystery of who we are by entering the void and the unknown, physical symptoms and illnesses will arise and persist. The purpose of these is to thrust us into the midst of that which we have been avoiding. This is because once we are diagnosed with a physical condition or illness, we are forced to embrace the unknown, as we do not know how severe our symptoms will become and how our illness will unfold.

The natural response of most to such a situation is fear. However, we can overcome this fear if we have the wisdom to realize that the illness is meant to teach us how to embrace the mystery of who we are and source our lives from the depths of the void.

Embracing the unknown is not something that can be practiced; it can only be experienced. Most people only get glimpses of the unknown and rarely abide in this space for more than a fleeting moment. Although there is no specific practice that can immerse you in the void, all other steps and practices that you have been doing up to this point have primed your inner world to embrace the unknown.

You need to shatter your limiting beliefs, burn through your unresolved emotions, unravel the stories you have created to justify where your life situation lies, raise your vibrational frequency and be in the flow in order to fully enter the void which is the source of all that is and the ground of all healing. Once your inner world has been primed through these practices, all you need is a nudge to fully embrace the mystery of who you are which is incomprehensible to the mind. This nudge is stillness.

Stillness is not a practice like meditation or yoga. It is a state of being in which you become fully aware of your true nature, which is pure emptiness. This is not meant to be a depressing thought but is meant to liberate you from the shackles of the illusory self in which most of humanity is immersed.

The illusory self is the false notion of the reality of your physical body, thoughts, emotions, and memories. These are certainly aspects of who you are, as I have discussed before, but only in a relative sense. In the absolute sense, we are the unknown, the void, or the emptiness that so many of us fear. This fear is driven by the illusory self, of which the ego is one aspect. The absolute essence of who we are can, therefore, be truly experienced through stillness.

I define stillness as dropping identification with anything you have ever identified with in your life. This includes your roles, identities, relationships, victories, defeats, and material possessions.

Now, let me make a clarification here. I am not implying that there is anything wrong with these aspects of our daily lives, because we all have physical bodies, are in relationships with others, and accumulate some material things in our lives. There is a difference between experiencing these things and completely identifying with them. It is through identification with these fleeting aspects of our lives that we experience suffering, which includes chronic disease.

So how do we practice stillness, which is the complete removal of identification with the illusory aspects of who we are?

First, we need to understand that there is a difference between stillness and presence. Presence is the art of living in the current moment and letting go of regrets over the past and worries about the future. You still experience thoughts, emotions, and life events but pass through them without letting them drag you out of the moment.

Stillness is a deeper level of being in which you realize that you are not in the world but the world is in you and passes through you. You are the movie projector, flashing images that are all the aspects of your physical life onto the canvas, the background on which your life unfolds. In a sense, you are the moment in which all of life unfolds, and this becomes not only a realization but your actual reality. Deep inner stillness is required to achieve such a realization.

Deep inner stillness is the state into which we are all born, and it is only our interaction with the physical world that takes us away from it. It is the state we experience in a deep sleep, but it can also be a part of our waking reality. It is simply a matter of a subtle shift in our awareness to get into the gap. We must focus on the space between each beat of our hearts, our thoughts, words, the space all around us, and the vastness of our inner space beyond our thoughts and emotions.

Every human being has a depth that is as profound as that of the universe. It is one of the greatest mysteries of life. When we plunge into these depths, we explore the unknown that exists both within and without. This is not about meditation but about a shift in our focus from the things that usually draw our attention in life to the gaps and the void that typify the unknown. It is this void from which everything in our manifest world arose, and it is to this source that we must return. Contemplate the true nature of your reality, which lies beyond form and non-form. Beyond matter and energy, beyond life and death, beyond victory and defeat, beyond ecstasy and despair lies the void from which all these things arise. The void is the core of the unknown and the source of fear for so many. The irony is that this void or the unknown, which instills fear in so many, is actually the only thing in the universe that absolutely exists. Everything else is a false illusion of reality not the essence of reality itself.

The void, which exists in the gaps in our lives, and appears to be unknowable, is actually nothing more than pure love. Love is the source and essence of all that is, has been and will be, and the only thing that separates us from this realization is the false illusion of reality, which life in the physical realm mires us with.

The love I am talking about is not the romantic love of human relationships, which is part of the false illusion of reality. It is the pure unadulterated love that brought the entire universe into existence because it knew that creation was the next step in its own evolution.

Love can only exist in a vacuum for so long before it must be expressed through form, although the form is only expression of love, not love itself. Every aspect of form, no matter how we perceive it, is a pure expression of love. How can I say this about such things as illness, pain, starvation, poverty, and other forms of suffering? The truth is that we cannot know love unless we know its opposite which is fear.

This is why we need to experience fear in all of its forms in order to know pure love. Fear takes the forms of greed, jealousy, hate, shame, grief, pain, and other forms of suffering. These must be experienced in order to have a context for experiencing pure, unconditional love, which is the nature of the void, stillness, and the unknown. This is why we should not curse but bless these so-called negative experiences that provide a frame of reference for knowing love, light and the Divine. They give us a context with which to embrace the unknown.

We have discussed fear in an earlier chapter, but it takes on a different meaning when it comes to facing and accepting the unknown. Fear, in this context, is essentially what the ego feels when we start to glimpse the reality of our true nature, which is sourced from the unknown. The ego fears its annihilation, but fails to understand that by realizing our true nature we integrate all aspects of who we are, including our ego, into our Higher Self. This is the essence of healing.

This also provides a frame of reference for all of our life experiences, which cannot be understood at the physical level alone but must be understood at the spiritual level. At the level of the soul, the full spectrum of human experience is necessary in order to realize the truth of who we are. Experience is our greatest teacher, and there is no experience or outcome, no matter how horrifying it may seem to the mind, that does not point us in the direction of realizing our Higher Self.

The problem is that the mind likes to categorize our experiences and give them labels. Once we label an experience, this creates a frame of reference with which to categorize all other experiences as our life situation unfolds, meaning that they are judged and not allowed to flower within so that our full being can shine forth.

This helps us understand the purpose of illness, which is to create a context in which to experience true health and healing. Illness, therefore, should be embraced and loved for the truth it reveals to us about the nature of healing.

Healing is not the absence of illness; it is the realization that illness is an aspect of our physical body that has separated from the whole and needs to be embraced and loved in order for us to reintegrate. This is where all true healing comes from. It lies deep inside that part of us we dare not enter for fear of losing our identity. Yet, we must plunge head first into that abyss, for it is the source of who we are: pure love.

In conclusion, you must embrace the unknown fully, regardless of your fear, in order to enter the void that is the source of your true love and nature, the root of all healing.

KEY POINTS

1. Embracing the unknown is the final step of the healing journey but the beginning of an infinite adventure into the depths of your being, which is as vast as the universe outside of you.
2. If you do not embrace the unknown, you will be forced to face it through the course of your illness.
3. Stillness is the medium through which the unknown can be embraced and explored.
4. The nature of the unknown or the void is simply pure love, which permeates the fabric of the universe.

5. Love can only exist in a vacuum for so long before it has to express itself in form through creation, which gives us a glimpse into the meaning of the universe.

QUESTIONS TO ASK YOUR CLIENTS

- Do you fear the unknown?
- Why do you fear the unknown?
- Do you think your fear is simply your ego fearing its loss of identity?
- Does your fear of the unknown have its source in your childhood fears of the dark and things you did not understand when you were younger?
- Have you ever been forced to face the unknown at any time in your life?
- If you were forced to face the unknown, what was the outcome?
- Did the outcome justify your fears?
- If the outcome did justify your fears, explain why?
- Did you come out of the situation unscathed?
- If you are still wearing the scars from that situation, what are they?
- How could embracing the unknown change your relationship with your illness?
- How could you cultivate a practice where you lean into the unknown on a regular basis?
- What does stillness mean to you?
- Do you practice stillness to any degree?
- How could you integrate stillness into your daily life?

CHAPTER 17

CREATION – MANIFESTING THE HEALTH YOU DESIRE

Once you have embraced the unknown, the source of all that is, and realized your true nature as love, then you are free to design your life and health as you desire. You can drop all negative habits, adopt excellent nutrition, and embrace movement and fitness as a natural extension of who you are.

These pursuits do not have to come from a place of motivation and willpower. On their own, they are not enough to change habits and behavior.

Why is this? Because the false sense must be convinced by motivation and willpower about what it needs to do to become happier and fulfilled. The problem, though, is that the false self can never be fulfilled; its nature is not your true nature, so this is impossible.

Once you drill down to the ground of your being and uncover your true nature, the false self slips away and is no longer a factor in designing the form that your outer life takes. This is because the false self becomes integrated into the whole of who you are and does not need to be convinced that it has to struggle to create the reality you desire.

This is why motivation and willpower are no longer factors in your external pursuits, as these now come straight from your source, your true nature, which is unveiled to you as you peel back the layers of what you are not. This is what we have been doing throughout this book.

Once our true nature is revealed to us, it becomes the source of manifestation in our lives. From our true nature, we are free to create our lives as we please, as we have been stripped free of all our blocks, so that the light of our being can shine forth from the depths of who we truly are.

This is how ultimate health is sourced and illness is transcended. You no longer seek the answers to your health from external sources; instead, the answers are revealed to you from the depths of your true nature, which is like a bright light illuminating everything in its path, including falsehood and illusion. If you were at one time dependent on medications, surgeries, or other external means to heal, your need for these modalities lessens over time. This is a gradual process as your true nature emerges from the ashes of who you once thought you were.

From this place of your essential self, you will intuitively know how much sleep your body needs, what specific nutritional needs your body has, and how much exercise and movement your body desires. You will instinctively avoid toxic habits that harm your body, such as tobacco, alcohol, and other addictions. If you have been in an abusive or toxic relationship, you will now naturally seek to end this disempowering union, which has been detrimental to your health. You will seek out the company of like-minded individuals who empower and uplift you.

You will attract circumstances in your life that will open you to new opportunities to expand your consciousness, your influence, and your financial abundance. You will soar where others only dream of flying. You will be a source of inspiration for others, who will seek to be in your glow and aspire to reach their own authenticity through your example. You will be a leader among leaders and show others how to heal with power and integrity. You will finally have come home.

When you finally arrive at this place, you realize yourself as the 99.99 percent of empty space, which is the true nature of the basic unit of matter, the atom. Once you see yourself as pure space and emptiness and not the illusion of a physical being, illness and disease no longer remain as major concerns; you realize that you are the source of your own health and can create your health as you desire.

Imagine the deep inner peace you would feel from this space. Imagine the freedom you would experience from knowing that you can engineer not only your health but your life as you desire. Imagine the comfort you would gain from knowing that your birth and death are only illusions of your physical body and not experiences of your true essence. Imagine the joy in realizing that no illness can come even close to touching the ground of your being, which is formless and timeless.

How can illness affect something that is formless? Imagine knowing yourself as formless, needless, loving, and infinite; a pure light in a time of darkness. This is what you experience as you peel back the layers of your false self and plunge into the depths of your inner being to unveil your true nature. This is the source of all creation in your physical reality, which includes optimal health and radical well-being.

KEY POINTS

1. Motivation and willpower are qualities that are needed to convince the false self of what it needs to do in order to become more happy and fulfilled.
2. Once you unveil your true nature, which is what the healing process is all about, everything you need to do to achieve optimal health, including the proper nutrition, the right amount of movement and exercise, and the right amount of sleep are sourced from your true nature and become a natural way of being rather than something that you have to achieve.
3. Once you unveil your true nature as formless and timeless, you realize that no illness can touch the ground of your being.

QUESTIONS TO ASK YOUR CLIENTS

(to be asked once they have completed the entire healing process)
*   What do you need to do in order to maintain your optimal health and well-being?

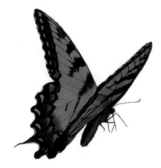

PART THREE

INTEGRATING AND
IMPLEMENTING
THE HEALING PROCESS

CHAPTER 18

A Diagnostic and Therapeutic Tool

The following list of questions is a diagnostic and therapeutic tool that you can use to help dive deep within to expose the roots of illness. It is simply a summary of all the questions at the ends of the previous chapters on the healing process.

As I have mentioned before, asking the right question can be transformational and dramatically change the course of your life. I encourage you to use this tool to help yourself and your patients and clients transform their health and their life situation once and for all.

- Have you ever set the intention to heal?
- If you did, were you able to follow through on your intention?
- If you were able to follow through on your intention, what was the outcome?
- If you were not able to follow through on your intention to heal, what do you think kept you from following through?
- What were your childhood dreams and ambitions?
- What have you enjoyed in the past or enjoy doing currently that keeps you so thoroughly engaged that you lose all track of time?
- What are your natural talents and abilities that you can perform effortlessly and that others complement you on?
- What brings joy, love, and peace to your life?
- Who are the people who you admire for their qualities, pursuits, and accomplishments?
- If you knew you could not fail, what would you attempt to do?
- What are some ways in which you could embody your connection to other people, nature, the earth, and the universe?
- What are the negative thoughts that sabotage your thinking?

- What are some positive thoughts that you could replace your negative thoughts with?
- How have your words hurt you or someone who you care about?
- Has this experience helped you realize the power of your words?
- What are some ways that you can encourage the people who you care about with your words?
- What is a universal healing mantra that you could use on a daily basis as a declaration to yourself and to the universe of your highest intention?
- What choices have you made or continue to make that keep you stuck in your comfort zone?
- How have these choices directed or limited your experience of life?
- What is the worst possible outcome if you were to lean outside your comfort zone?
- Could this worse possible outcome hurt or harm you in any permanent way?
- What is one simple thing you could do right now to lean outside your comfort zone?
- Can you identify your limiting beliefs through your negative thought patterns and personal challenges? Make a list of them.
- Ask yourself if these limiting beliefs hold any validity?
- Can you find evidence to prove that your limiting beliefs are not true?
- Can you find an alternate meaning to your limiting beliefs?
- Can you reframe your limiting beliefs into empowering beliefs?
- How can you embody your newly formed empowering beliefs?
- What are the recurrent emotional patterns in your life that keep you stuck and prevent you reaching your full potential?
- Can you trace a recurrent emotional pattern back to the sentinel event that birthed it?
- If you cannot trace a recurrent emotional pattern back to the sentinel event, where do you feel these emotions in your body?
- If you were to experience the emotions around the sentinel event to their fullest extent, what is the worst thing that could happen to you?

- How would your life transform if you were able to burn through your unresolved emotions fully and experience the peace at their core?
- What is keeping you from burning through your unresolved emotions and releasing them once and for all?
- Can you recall some milestones in your life where you felt fear?
- Did you take action despite the fear?
- If you did, what was the outcome?
- If you didn't, what possible outcomes did you deprive yourself of?
- What in your life currently causes you fear?
- What is this fear telling you about the direction you must take?
- What could be the greatest possible outcome from making the choice that is causing you fear?
- What are the stories that you have created to perpetuate your chronic illness?
- Is there any validity or truth to your stories?
- Is there any evidence you can find to dismantle the stories you have created around your illness?
- If you were to dismantle the stories you have created around your chronic disease, what would it mean for your overall health?
- Who would you be without your life story?
- Can you trace a pattern through all of your past and current life experiences?
- Does this pattern reveal anything to you about your life's greater mission?
- If this pattern does not reveal to you your life's mission, then what are the missing pieces that could lead you to the truth of why you are here?
- How would discovering your life's greater mission transform your experience of life?
- What is the fundamental nature of who you truly are?
- Is your current nutrition supporting your highest vibrational frequency?
- If not, then what changes could you make in your nutritional choices to increase your vibrational frequency?
- Are there any addictive substances or activities you are engaged in that are lowering your vibrational frequency?

- How can you truly break free of these addictions?
- How can you experience joy in every moment of your life?
- What can you do to express the love that you are?
- What are you grateful for in this very moment?
- Can you find something to be grateful for every day of your life?
- What are some of the things that you appreciate in your life?
- Are you able to appreciate your personal challenges by allowing them to reveal their deeper purpose in your life?
- How would your experience of life transform if you were to find a way to appreciate your life's personal challenges?
- Do you remember a time when you were completely in the flow?
- Do you remember what you were thinking, how you felt, and what you were focusing on in the moment that you were in the flow?
- Can you see that flow is the natural state of your body's physiology and is essential for your optimal health?
- What are some of the ways in which you could embody flow in your life?
- How would your life transform if you were to see everyone and everything around you as simply an extension of yourself?
- How would you integrate these practices to enter the flow into your daily life?
- How can you consistently get into and stay in the zone?
- How would being in the flow transform your relationships with those closest to you, your immediate environment, the world at large?
- How would our world transform if more and more people were consistently in the flow?
- Do you fear the unknown?
- Why do you fear the unknown?
- Do you think your fear is simply your ego fearing its loss of identity?
- Does your fear of the unknown have its source in your childhood fears of the dark and things you did not understand when you were younger?
- Have you ever been forced to face the unknown at any time in your life?
- If you were forced to face the unknown, what was the outcome?
- Did the outcome justify your fears?

- If the outcome did justify your fears, explain why?
- Did you come out of the situation where you were forced to face the unknown unscathed?
- If you are still wearing the scars from that situation, what are they?
- How could embracing the unknown change your relationship with your illness?
- How could you cultivate a practice where you lean into the unknown on a regular basis?
- What does stillness mean to you?
- Do you practice stillness to any degree?
- How could you integrate stillness into your daily life?
- What do you need to do in order to maintain your optimal health and well-being?

KEY POINTS

1. Asking the right questions is the key to engaging the healing process.
2. If you dive deep into the questions presented in this diagnostic and therapeutic tool, your path to healing will unfold naturally.

CHAPTER 19

THE ROLE OF
CONVENTIONAL MEDICINE

We have just completed a journey from illusion to reality, from false-hood to truth, from the external to the internal, from the multiple roles we play in our physical lives to the essence of who we truly are.

The problem is that, even after having read to this point in this book, most people will not have had the realizations that I have been discussing. To peel back the layers of the false self is, for most people, a lifelong journey, with gradual progress over time, and does not happen at the pace of this book. This also means that everyone is at different stages in their healing journey.

This is why conventional medical treatments, such as medications and surgery, are needed for most people, and for this reason, my book is not about ending the use of modern medicine. Quite the contrary: this book wholly embraces these treatments as necessary at various stages of the healing journey.

The other important realization we all eventually have is that we are not just physical beings but are mental, emotional, vibrational, and spiritual beings. Whatever ails the physical self often begins at deeper levels of our being and is often a wakeup call for us to realize these deeper aspects of who we are. If you do not heed this call, or begin the healing journey and do not fully complete it, the physical condition will progress over time, as it has not fully served its purpose of taking you deeper into the depths of who you truly are.

As the physical body deteriorates, the unveiling process may or may not occur but inevitably occurs as we approach death. Death is the stripping away of everything that is not real, leaving us as the pure essential self we were before we were born into physical form.

This is why the death of a loved one is not to be mourned but to be cherished for the truth of what it is, although we can mourn our own loss of that loved one. This is even true of the death of children, as they are closer to their true nature and have less fear than their adult counterparts who usually experience physical deterioration and death with much fear and trepidation.

As a critical care and palliative care specialist, I have witnessed the deaths of hundreds of patients, and in almost all cases, before death, patients reach a point where they are overcome with a profound peace. This can be seen in their facial expressions, even if they are comatose. I believe that all dying patients who experience this transition realize the true nature of their being, even if they lived their lives in falsehood, attached and addicted to their physical nature. I believe that this change in a dying patient's demeanor is also meant to bring comfort to the loved ones who are left behind, who often do not realize this when I interact with them.

In essence, death is the stripping away of all that is not real and the unveiling of our true nature. I am not implying that death should be accepted and welcomed as inevitable, if there are options for treatment of the patient. However, there are situations in which, despite all treatment, patients will deteriorate because they are nearing the end of their lives. In these situations, death becomes the ultimate healing, as the physical is stripped away and all that remains is the patient's true spiritual essence. This has profound implications for the practice of hospice and palliative care medicine, which could be transformed by these realizations and bring peace and comfort to the thousands of family members who face the death of a loved one every day.

The problem with conventional medicine is not its role in the treatment of chronic disease. We have already established that these treatments are needed for most people in modern society who do not have the wisdom or the courage to dive deeply enough to start unveiling their true essence. The issue is that conventional medicine keeps patients locked in the paradigm of dependence on physical treatments without providing a path for exploration of why they have become ill and what can be done about this at an existential level.

The role of our healthcare system should be to help patients heal at a deeper level, but this is not what is happening. We have created a "disease care" system that keeps patients trapped in a paradigm of remaining sick, depending on medications and invasive procedures, and often ending up hospitalized. Patients then become locked in a vicious cycle of suffering from the symptoms of chronic disease with little relief from medications, cycling between physician's offices, emergency departments, inpatient hospital wards and, often, intensive care units.

This is not what the healthcare system was meant to be. It was meant to be a source of solace, comfort, and healing; instead, it has become a means of perpetuating pain and suffering for patients and families.

I envision a healthcare system where the goal is to heal and to not solely justify its existence by ensuring its profits through perpetuating chronic disease. I envision a healthcare system where patients do get the usual physical treatments they need but are then facilitated in a process of deeper healing. I envision patients being introduced to the process of healing I have introduced in this book.

I realize that not all patients will be ready to take the deep dive within that is necessary to fully heal, but it is an injustice to not offer patients the option of a path to true healing. I am not suggesting that the process in this book is the only path to healing; however, any process used must address mindset, emotions, energy, flow, and spirit or consciousness. It is only through accessing deeper levels of being that one can be truly healed.

This will require a new breed of healthcare practitioners of the inner realms and a new psychology of healing. Most hospitals offer spiritual care in the form of chaplains and pastors, but their role is only to provide comfort to patients and their families. What I am proposing is a complete overhaul of our healthcare system to provide physical, mental, emotional, vibrational, and spiritual healing.

I believe that the time is right for such a revolution in healthcare. Having worked in healthcare for twenty years at the time of this book being published, I have witnessed the disillusionment of patients firsthand. I have witnessed their pain and suffering every day. I also have witnessed the emotional turmoil brought upon their families by their loved one's suffering. I believe that patients and their families are ready for a new paradigm in healthcare. They are ready for the healthcare system to live up to its promise of being the sanctuary of healing it was always meant to be. The time to take back your health is now.

KEY POINTS

- Because most people will be at various stages in their healing journey, the majority will require conventional medical care to some degree as part of their healing process.
- Death is the stripping away of all that is not real and remains the final healing gateway for all, even if they have identified with illusion and falsehood throughout their entire lives.
- The healthcare system needs to change and embrace a greater healing paradigm, as outlined in this book.

CHAPTER 20

THE PATH TO CHANGE

The path to change begins with each of us as individuals. We have to realize that we have been living an illusion of the physical being the only aspect of who we are. We need to realize that we are more than our bodies and must start to embody the deeper levels of our being. We must also begin treating others as the multidimensional beings that they are and realize that we are not separate from one another. We are all connected at the deepest level of energy and spirit and are all part of the universal consciousness. Even if you do not engage in the process outlined in this book, I encourage you to seek more holistic means of healing beyond conventional treatments. These may include meditation in all of its various forms, yoga, qigong, conscious breathing, energy healing methods, herbalism, nutritional therapy, and a host of other methods now available to us.

Each of these practices fits into the framework of healing that I have presented in this book. Mindfulness and meditation are practices of inner flow; yoga and qigong are practices of body flow; and conscious breathing is a practice of physiologic flow. Energy healing, herbalism, and nutritional therapy are all modalities that raise your personal vibrational frequency. So, although you may not want to engage in the process I have outlined in this book in its entirety, you must realize that any healing modality that exists in the world today is only a part of this greater framework of healing as discussed in this book. Even if you do not engage in the entire process, any of these modalities can begin to facilitate the process of true inner healing which will permeate outward to the physical body.

It is not enough for us to engage inner self-healing individually but to educate and coach others close to us, such as our family, friends, acquaintances, and co-workers. This knowledge needs to spread like wildfire to as many people as possible to create a threshold for massive social and, eventually, global change in how we approach our health.

As this deeper healing knowledge becomes revealed to more and more people, we will begin to see more awareness of this in social media, which is a huge catalyst of change. There will likely be resistance in the mainstream media, as this is usually controlled by large corporate interests whose profit in some way is generally tied to the disease care system.

Examples of these large corporate interests are large fast food chains, processed food companies, pharmaceutical companies, medical device companies, and any company connected to the sugar industry, to name a few. When profits are at stake, resistance to change is inevitable and unavoidable. However, despite these fears, our mainstream media must be infiltrated and true deeper healing must be promoted if we are to be bold enough to dare to transform the health of the general population.

This can be done in many ways. The first thing is to identify individuals you know who are suffering from chronic disease. This is not hard to do, given the state of health of the average person in the general population.

Once you have identified one person, or several people, ask them how they are doing. How are they managing? How are their symptoms? How many medications do they take? Have they suffered any complications or side effects from their medications? Have they had to have any surgeries? Have they had complications from any surgical procedures? Are they happy with their current medical care? Could their health be improved in any way? Have they tried any other means beyond conventional medicine to heal their condition?

Even if their condition is being managed effectively, and they are happy with their care, you can ask them other questions. How much do their medications cost them monthly? Would they be happier if they were dependent on fewer medications? How is their emotional health? Do they feel deeply connected to themselves to others and nature? Do they often get anxious or depressed? Do they lament over the past or worry about the future? Are they under undue stress? How do they handle stress in their lives? What are their coping strategies? Have they succumbed to stress at any time in the past or recently? Are they able to genuinely relax, have fun, and enjoy their lives, despite what is happening in their life situation?

Somewhere in the midst of this questioning, you will likely be able to find an opening in the individual's responses where the concepts introduced in this book can be of tremendous benefit. The point is to get the person thinking introspectively and to go deeper within, to the root of their physical or emotional health issues. It is only there that they will find the answers they are seeking.

Once you are able to get a few individuals talking and thinking about their health in a new light, you can then form meetup or discussion groups where these ideas can be openly discussed in a public forum. You may want to start with a small committed group of individuals and then expand this group to include more and more people who could benefit through word of mouth. You will likely generate so much interest in this process of healing that you will have to break your meeting into smaller groups that meet regularly to discuss and engage in the process.

You may even want to take your group online in the form of a blog, an online meetup, or a Facebook group to engage a wider audience in the healing dialogue. You will then be able to reach beyond your immediate geography and engage individuals in other countries and continents to spread this message further.

As the popularity of deeper healing through unveiling your true nature grows, the popular media must be actively engaged to help spread this message. They will likely initially be resistant, because they usually latch onto sensational or sexy topics, which this is not. However, they will not be able to avoid this topic once they see its effects on people's health and chronic disease.

This is why we must actively engage the media in promoting deeper levels of healing through the unveiling process and other means mentioned earlier. This can be done by writing letters to local newspapers, calling in to local radio shows, and pressuring local news stations to air stories related to healing, as we have been discussing.

In addition to engaging popular media, you must engage social media to exponentially educate as many people as possible about the path to true healing. This can be done through Facebook and LinkedIn posts and sending tweets about how to truly heal. As noted above, you can also create a blog or a Facebook group about healing and start to discuss the concepts you have learned in this book.

This kind of open online discussion is a great way to introduce these healing concepts to those who may not be fully ready to commit to this healing path. The key is to help people understand that there is more to health and healing than just the physical treatments they are used to and to introduce them to the deeper aspects of healing as discussed in this book.

As inner healing gains more popularity on social media, and in the online world in general, you will be able to generate enough publicity and attention to these issues that interest in them will grow exponentially and, crucially, generate a lot of online noise. This is essential in order to create enough momentum to shift public attitudes and beliefs regarding health and healing and ignite the spark of change in our healthcare system, the ultimate goal. This is the path to change in today's healthcare system.

KEY POINTS

1. The path to changing the overall health of the general population and the healthcare system begins with each of us as individuals, if we are committed to seeing this change in our lifetimes.
2. In order to change the health of the general population and transform our global healthcare systems, we have to engage various means of spreading the message of true healing, including our immediate circle of influence and social and mainstream media.

CHAPTER 21

Beyond Health

The process I have introduced in this book is not just applicable to health and healing; it can also transform our relationships, our careers, our wealth consciousness, and our overall freedom.

For example, limiting beliefs do not just apply to our health but can apply to our relationships and attitudes to wealth.

Some limiting beliefs about relationships include: I will never find love, I will never get along with my partner, I will never get over my last breakup, I will never be happy in a relationship, I am meant to be alone, I am unlovable, and I have too much pain to love another person.

Some limiting beliefs about wealth include: my parents were poor so I am always destined to be poor, I will always be stuck in my dead end job, I will never get out of debt, I need a higher degree in order to know how to successfully run a business, I will never be a successful entrepreneur, and I will never be financially free.

Emotional blocks can also be detrimental to all aspects of our lives. We all create stories around our interactions and connections with others, namely our relationships, the source of much drama in many people's lives.

Not being in the flow can affect how our relationships flow and the flow of abundance and wealth into our lives. Fear of the unknown and not openly embracing the unknown can keep us from our true potential, not only in our health but also in the richness of our relationships and in our true wealth potential.

As you can see, this healing process is widely applicable to all areas of your life and should be utilized wherever you need it at this moment. Let the moment guide you where you will go and then dive deeply into the healing process.

So where is this all going? The healing process is meant to take you to a place of freedom—freedom from the symptoms of chronic disease; freedom from relationship fatigue, tension, and drama; freedom from the feeling of financial lack; and spiritual freedom for your soul to soar to unlimited heights.

This freedom can only come from diving deeply into the vastness of your true nature and exploring it with pure abandon. This is what the healing process, as outlined in this book, is all about.

The healing process is also crucial to alleviating the stress response, which, if left unabated, can lead to immune dysfunction and chronic disease. Stress itself is not the issue; it is the body's response to stress that is the problem. We live in a society in which stress is the norm of daily life. Our lives have become complicated because of more demanding jobs, more pressure on our children to excel in both academics and extracurricular activities, technology that increases demands on our attention and makes the demands of our bosses, our families, and friends instantaneous, and numerous other factors.

As outlined earlier, our adrenal glands secrete the hormone cortisol in response to chronic stress. Cortisol normally suppresses inflammation, but if cortisol is present for long periods of time, the body develops cortisol resistance, which increases the production of pro-inflammatory substances, called cytokines. This leads to a state of chronic inflammation and the development of chronic inflammatory and autoimmune conditions, such as heart disease, diabetes mellitus, cancer, dementias such as Alzheimer's disease, and connective tissue diseases such as rheumatoid arthritis, to name a few.

Prolonged increased cortisol secretion associated with chronic stress also lowers the amounts of proteins in the body, which are critical for signaling other immune cells, and suppresses lymphocytes, which increases the risk of acute infection.

The healing process can help us navigate stress through many means. Eliminating our limiting beliefs around stress and replacing them with empowering beliefs can give us tremendous advantages when it comes to dealing with the stresses of daily life. Removing emotional blocks can alleviate negative emotional responses to stressful circumstances and allow us to approach these with a more holistic perspective. Raising our personal vibrational level and getting in the flow can allow us to navigate stressful situations in our lives with greater ease. Embracing the unknown can essentially nullify the ill effects of stress in our lives by giving us a mechanism to manage fear of the unknown as I have discussed earlier, which is a major cause of stress for most. Therefore, true healing is essential to effectively managing the stress that has become the norm in today's fast-paced society.

The healing process, as I have described in this book, should be an essential part of our education system. It can teach our children critical coping mechanisms for managing stress, preventing illness, and how to live their lives to the fullest. The problem with our schools, as noted earlier, is that they teach facts and figures but do not teach what really matters: how to live life with peace, passion, meaning, and purpose.

The healing journey is directly applicable to health and healing but can also help children find inner peace. Once they are able to do that, no matter their external circumstances, a space opens up inside them. This space creates a place for their passion to be slowly kindled and ignited into a raging fire, which leads them in the direction of discovering their life's mission.

Imagine if every child had the opportunity to find inner peace and discover what they are truly passionate about. Imagine every child being able to reach their highest potential. Imagine what this would do for their emotions, their confidence, and their conviction. Imagine the creativity that would emerge from such an environment and how it could fuel solutions to the world's greatest problems. Imagine success being defined not by testing and grades but by whether a child has discovered their true passion and is on the path to discovering their life's mission. Imagine how this would transform the educational atmosphere into a place of pure, unbridled joy.

Even though our schools are probably not ready to introduce such a radical idea into their curricula, it is important to teach your children this entire process as early as they are able to comprehend it. This need not be complicated but can be adjusted to a child's understanding. This is what I'll discuss in the next chapter.

KEY POINTS

1. The healing process is not only applicable to health but can transform any area of life including your relationships, your financial abundance, your response to stress, and your sense of personal and spiritual freedom, to name a few.
2. The healing process should be interwoven into the education of our children, who only serve to benefit from it.

CHAPTER 22

The Healing Process
For Children

The application of the healing process to children is subtly different than that I have described for adults, since for children, I eliminate the steps of exploration and creation. The reason I do this is because, by simplifying the process, it makes it more likely that children will engage in it. We can discuss embracing the unknown at the end of the process, and it does not need to be repeated at the beginning through exploration. I eliminate the last step of creation, since it is usually directed by their parents and need not be assigned to the children themselves.

As children grow older, the step of creation will become more relevant to them, as they will become mature enough to manifest the health they desire.

The healing process for children therefore becomes:

1. Intention
2. Mentation
3. Emotion
4. Narration
5. Vibration
6. Motion
7. Exploration

I would like to discuss each of these in some detail as they apply to children. First, intention needs to be simplified for children. Depending on their age and understanding, children may not be able to comprehend the concept of "setting an intention to heal." Even if they do not suffer from illness, they may need to heal from stress, anxiety, depression, or early childhood trauma. The problem is that they may not understand this. We need to ask children a different question.

In the chapter on intention, I discussed finding your "powerful why." But you cannot ask children this question, because they may not be able to give a sophisticated answer. As far as they're concerned, they simply get up in the morning because they have to, not because they have a powerful reason to. So the question you must ask the child is what—*what* do you love to do so much that you could do it all day long?

You cannot accept mundane answers to this question, such as watching television, playing video games, or playing with friends. A child must be encouraged to dig deep enough to reveal to himself or herself what he or she loves to do, then this powerful what becomes the basis of their intention to heal. It could be drawing, playing a specific sport, reading books, learning at school, helping their grandparents, connecting with nature, or a host of other things. But it must be discovered so that it can form the basis for the child's intention to heal.

Now, I realize that not every child will know what their powerful what is. This is why children should be encouraged to safely explore their interests as fully as possible in order to discover where their passions lie and where their talents can be cultivated. It is only through helping children discover their powerful what that you will be able to ignite in them a fire that not only heals them but sparks their passion, purpose, success, and fulfillment.

The next step is to identify the child's limiting beliefs. Usually, children have not had enough life experience to have developed limiting beliefs but, if present, they must be identified. One way to do this is to ask the child if there is anything he believes that he cannot accomplish. If the child does identify something, then it is your job to eliminate and replace this with an empowering belief. This can be done by first finding the source of the limiting belief.

For example, if the child feels that he cannot be a great basketball player, it may be because he once played on his schoolyard with his friends and did not play very well. It could also be that he tried out for the school team and did not make it. You may not find a source of the limiting belief, in which case it becomes easier to remove it. However, if you do find a source, then you need to determine its validity in the child's eyes.

For example, if the child only played basketball a few times or only tried out once for the team, you can point out that it takes hours and hours of practice and dedication to make him into a great basketball player, so his limiting belief around being a bad player holds no validity. You can give examples to the child where this limiting belief is not true, a perfect example being the fact that the greatest player who played in the NBA, Michael Jordan, was cut from his high school basketball team at one time.

You can then help him reframe the limiting belief. For example, the fact that he did not make the basketball team the first time he tried out is a sign that he needs to practice more and improve his skills. You then replace the limiting belief with an empowering belief. In this example, this can be, "I am a great basketball player and can play amongst the best players anywhere." You have the child reinforce this belief while developing irrefutable proof that this is true through practice and dedication to improving his skills.

The same principles can be applied to any limiting belief. For any limiting belief, it is important that you develop this irrefutable proof that the new empowering belief is true because children are very intelligent. If they do not see proof of what they are being told, this will create an inner conflict, which will create fear, doubt, and mistrust and could lead to more problems for the child.

The next step is to eliminate any emotional blocks. Children are usually not old enough to have developed these emotional blocks but, for those who have had early traumatic childhood experiences, these may be present.

Even if the child has had no traumatic experiences, the experience of birth—leaving the mother's womb and entering the physical world—is traumatic for everyone, as I have already discussed in an earlier chapter. The baby is essentially being taken out of a place of safety and comfort and thrust into the unknown realm of the physical world of which they have no prior experience.

It may not be wise to ask a child to experience the emotions around a prior traumatic experience, as can be done for adults. The reason for this is that the response that a child will have to experiencing painful emotions is unpredictable, since the child may not be mature enough to differentiate the emotion from the experience or situation that caused the emotion, especially if the situation is no longer actively affecting the child.

This being the case, every child's situation must be judged individually as to whether they can handle experiencing trapped emotions from the past to their fullest extent. What children can be taught is to feel their emotions fully and deeply and to not hold them back in the moment that they are experienced in a socially conscious way. This can be done in a protective environment around people that they trust such as their parents, older siblings, other relatives, close friends, teachers, and so forth.

Children are closer to their true nature and are generally more apt to be honest with their feelings, so they usually do not need a lot of encouragement. What they do need is a safe haven or space in order to express their feelings, and it is the job of all responsible, compassionate, and caring adults to provide this container for children to express fully and deeply.

This can be encouraged by regularly talking to them about their day-to-day experiences and how they made them feel. Children must also be encouraged to express how they feel in the moment, even if the feelings are sadness, fear, anger, bitterness, or rage. Feelings that are not expressed and experienced fully will become trapped somewhere in the child's subconscious mind and, eventually, will manifest in the body as physical symptoms that could potentially evolve into an illness. This is why children must be taught uninhibited, free expression of their deepest emotions so they can be released to unveil what lies beneath, their true nature.

The next step in the healing process for children is that of narration. Usually, children have not accumulated much in the way of life stories that they identify with but some may have. However, most children have not lived long enough to develop a life story that they use to justify their illness if they suffer from one. Even if they are not ill, this step is crucial to their maturation and growth into an adult, because it can provide clarity as to their life's path. What children should be encouraged to do is to tell their stories from their day and to journal about them as soon as they are able to write. They should then be encouraged to extract what they learned from this story.

This is important because by getting their story out in the open and sharing it with an adult, it is less likely that they will end up identifying with it and more likely that they will be able to gain the lesson in their story. If they journal about their stories, over time they will have an accumulated narrative. An important adult in the child's life can help them trace a common thread through this narrative by identifying common patterns in their stories.

As the child gets older and enters adolescence and early adulthood, they can use the common thread or patterns they have identified to draw out their life's mission as an expression of their higher purpose. This will ensure the child's happiness and success in life, as true happiness and success come from being part of something greater than yourself, namely your life's mission. This is why it is important to encourage children to express their stories and journal about them on a regular basis.

The next step is to help raise the child's vibrational frequency. Children are usually in a higher state of vibration than adults, since they are closer to their true nature of unconditional love and joy. What you, as an adult, can do is to reinforce those feelings at every moment possible. You must bring out the child's natural state of love by reflecting their love back to them. This is done by giving them undivided focused attention when they are in your presence.

This is hard to do in the busy, multitasking, and distracted lifestyle that most people live today. However, it is vital to the child's development that they have all of your attention, for even a few minutes, when they are in your presence. This reinforces to them their importance in your eyes and is a manifestation of your love for them, which brings out their natural state of unconditional love.

It is also important to bring out the child's joy by being joyful in their presence. I know that this is often challenging when you are dealing with ongoing daily issues at work, in your relationships, in your health, and in your home, but its importance cannot be overemphasized. There are few things that are as damaging to a child than an adult's negativity. Even if you are dealing with challenges in your daily life, this does not prevent you from sharing a smile, some stories, and even a good laugh with your child.

You should teach your children gratitude, to be grateful for even the simplest things in their lives. You should ask your children at the dinner table or before they go to sleep what they are grateful for today and encourage them to journal about their gratitude daily. It is also vital to appreciate your children at every possible opportunity. Try to see the good that they do, regardless of the situation, and encourage them at every step of their lives, even if they falter or fall short of your expectations. You must remember that you were also once a struggling child, trying to discover who you are and trying to find your way in the world.

If I were to summarize these recommendations in a nutshell, I would say that you should hug and kiss your children at least daily, if not more often; encourage them to share their stories of the day; smile and laugh with them often; encourage them to express daily gratitude; and show appreciation for at least one thing they tried or accomplished every day. These practices will go a long way to helping to raise your children's vibration.

After a child is anchored in a high state of vibration, it does not take much to get them into a state of flow. Children, naturally, live in the moment and therefore are always in a state of flow until adults interfere with their demands and expectations. Therefore, it is crucial for adults to let children live in the moment, as they naturally do, with little interference.

Now, this does not mean that they do not occasionally need some direction to get up in the morning for school, to do their homework, to get involved in extracurricular activities, and to be disciplined for ill behavior. Direction and encouragement is a necessary part of any child's development; however, this should be the exception and not the norm.

To keep a child in a state of flow, you can apply some of the same practices that we discussed earlier in the chapter on flow. Children can be mentored in inner flow by teaching them to focus on their thoughts and emotions, no matter what they are, without judging them and to talk about them if they feel impelled to.

They can be mentored in physiologic flow by showing them the rhythm of their heartbeat and pulse and teaching them that these signify the flow of blood throughout their circulatory system to all the different organs, tissues, and cells of their body. Physiologic flow can also be reinforced by teaching children to focus on the inflow and outflow of their breath without altering it. They can be taught that the flow of air into the lungs delivers oxygen to the bloodstream and to all the cells of the body through the circulation. Body flow is something that children naturally manifest, since they are usually active and moving most of the time.

Outer flow in the world can be mentored by revealing to children that their entire world is just an extension of them, and that there is no separation between them, other people, and everything they can perceive with their five senses. Even though they may not fully understand this concept, it must still be introduced early on, in order for it to become planted and germinate in their consciousness.

Outer flow in the world can also be mentored in children by having them spend more time in nature so that they can experience, firsthand, the interconnection and interdependence among trees, plants, insects, birds, animals, ponds, rivers and lakes, and weather patterns. Children should experience the sheer beauty of the natural world in all its glory and manifestation to see how it flows effortlessly in cycles. These practices will help keep children in a state of flow, which is vital for emotional and physical health.

The final step in the unveiling process is to help children embrace the unknown. Children are naturally more prone to embrace the unknown than adults because they have less fear and more curiosity than adults. It does not take much to take a child down this path, but a continuous curiosity and love for trying new and different things must be cultivated in the child if they are to have an engaging relationship with the void. This can be done by exposing the child to various new pursuits in different fields of athletics, intellect, music, art, community service, and anything they feel drawn to, as long as it is relatively safe.

Children should be encouraged to try new and different pursuits, and this does not have to be a costly undertaking. Children's curiosity can be cultivated through free and unstructured play in a natural setting where they are free to explore nature in all her wonderful glory. Nature is a field of infinite discovery where one is always engaging with the unknown and learning new things. In addition, studies have shown that spending time in nature stimulates the intellect, calms the mind, and increases positive emotions.

Children should also be taught the power of choice and how this faculty lays out the path they will be following in life. Children should be taught to make safe and healthy choices but also to make choices that take them outside their comfort zone. You can help children step outside their comfort zones by being there with them in the early stages of their engagement with the unknown, to show them that they are more capable and courageous than they previously thought.

This could be simply trying a new activity or sport, making a new friend at a playground, or making their first purchase at a store. By cultivating a child's healthy relationship with the unknown, you will teach them to continually push the limits of their comfort zone despite fear. This will get the child more in touch with the source of their existence and unlimited potential and, thus, the source of all healing.

KEY POINTS

- The healing process is as vital for children as it is for adults and can be engaged at any age and at any stage in their development.

CHAPTER 23

Why Seek Healing Versus Cure?

Why seek healing and not cure, you may ask? This is a very important question and needs to be discussed in the proper context.

When most people think about cure, they are referring to a result at the level of the physical body that equates to a complete removal of the condition they are suffering from. The problem with seeking a cure is that it only refers to the dimension of the physical body; it does not address the many layers that define who we are.

I have already discussed that you are a multidimensional being, with mental, emotional, vibrational, spiritual, and existential aspects to yourself. Healing refers to the process of becoming whole, which means to integrate all the various aspects of your being to create the highest expression of who you are. This is the process that I have been outlining throughout this book.

This is important because what manifests in the physical body is often a result of issues at different levels of our being. One may argue that disease occurs as a result of a complex interplay between our genetics and our environment. However, epigenetics is a more powerful determinant of health than genetics alone, as mentioned earlier in this book. Epigenetics refers to how the environment in which you are brought up affects the expression of your genetic blueprint, that is, switches on or off genes that may lead to the development of chronic disease.

It is not simply the environment that affects your genetic expression but how you respond to your environment. Your response to your environment is conditioned by your subconscious mind, your emotional self, your vibrational frequency, and, ultimately, your spiritual self. The development of illness, thus, ties back to the higher aspects of your being, which is why healing is a more comprehensive and holistic approach to dealing with disease than simply seeking a cure.

Let's discuss this in the context of a condition that is on the rise and affects millions of people around the world: cancer.

There is no debating the fact that cancer is a devastating disease, which can affect almost any organ system in the body. The five-year survival rates for various cancers vary from 17 percent for lung cancer to 64 percent for colorectal cancer to 88 percent for breast cancer.[1] Survival rates depend on the extent of the cancer at the time of diagnosis and tend to be worse when diagnosed in later stages. In fact, in 2011, almost 30 percent of all deaths in Canada were due to cancer.

But what really is cancer? Cancer is defined as an uncontrolled division and growth of abnormal cells in a part of the body. Over time, cancer cells start to affect and, eventually, take over the normal functioning of the organ in which they manifest. The traditional approach to cancer treatment has been either to hack it out (surgery), poison it out (chemotherapy), or burn it out (radiation therapy). These approaches are often effective initially but, in many cases, do not result in a definite cure.

The term remission is used frequently among cancer specialists, but it only means that the physical exam, blood tests, and radiologic scans show that all signs of your cancer are gone. Physicians will tell you that this does not equate to cure. In fact, many cancers recur within five years of the last treatment.

So why are conventional treatments often ineffective over time? And is cancer simply a disease of the physical body?

As a pulmonologist, I have diagnosed many patients with lung cancer, and as a critical care specialist, I often see patients with other types of cancer with acute and serious complications. In almost all of the cases of cancer I have diagnosed and treated, there was not one patient who did not suffer from one or a combination of the following: limiting beliefs, emotional blocks, negative attitudes leading to a low vibrational frequency, feeling like they were stuck somewhere in their lives and therefore out of the flow, debilitating fear of the unknown that kept them stuck in their comfort zones, or other deep existential issues.

This suggests that cancer is not just a disease of the physical body but begins at deeper levels of one's being and, over time, eventually manifests in the physical body. Cancer can, therefore, be seen as an emotional, vibrational, or existential disease. This is why conventional treatments alone are often ineffective in completely curing cancer to the point that even cancer specialists will never tell you that you are cured but simply in remission.

Conventional treatments do not take into account the deeper issues of one's being that need to be addressed, as I have been discussing throughout this book. It is only by navigating these deeper issues with unswerving resolve that you can truly heal and, potentially, cure yourself of cancer.

I have been using cancer as an example, but this can apply to any chronic disease process that you suffer from. All chronic diseases have their roots in deeper aspects of our being, and the physical body is simply the final place where they manifest. This is the main point of this book.

KEY POINTS

1. Cure only refers to the dimension of the physical body and does not address the multidimensional nature of who you are, which includes your mental, emotional, vibrational, spiritual, and existential self.

2. Healing refers to the process of becoming whole, which means to integrate all the various aspects of your being to create the highest expression of who you are.

CHAPTER 24

IS IT NOT TOO DIFFICULT
TO HEAL?

You may be thinking that the path to healing is too complex and difficult to navigate, and I would not disagree with you. Excavating the deeper dimensions of your being takes effort and is not for the faint of heart.

However, if you are wondering whether it is worth the effort, then I would simply ask you some questions. Is it worth foregoing the effort to do some inner work to spend your life suffering with the effects of chronic disease and to have no control over your health? Is it better to be at the mercy of the many thousands of illnesses that can befall you? Are you willing to let chronic disease derail you from success in other areas of your life, such as your relationships, your finances, your life's mission, and your spiritual goals? Are you willing to live your life far below your true potential, never experiencing the possibilities that lie just beyond your reach?

One of the founding fathers of the United States, Thomas Jefferson, once said that if you want something you've never had, you've got to do something you've never done. This applies as much to healing as it does to anything else in life. It is true that there is effort involved in walking the path to true healing, and it is often a daunting and arduous road. However, the rewards for taking this journey are immeasurable, and what lies on the other side is indescribable. This is truly a journey of a lifetime as you peel back the layers of illusion of who you think you are to reveal the truth and the depth of your true nature. The beauty of this exploration into consciousness is that it is without destination, as it is infinite and reveals more of its brilliance as you plunge further into its depths.

So to answer the question that began this chapter, yes, healing is usually an arduous road that forces you to face your deeper fears and inner demons. However, if you have the courage to take this journey and simply be open to everything that you encounter along the way, you will find that a lot of what scares you is simply an illusion. You will also find immeasurable rewards, as I have already mentioned, which take the effort of confronting your deepest fears in order for them to be revealed to you. Confronting these deep fears is akin to the effort required to achieve other difficult goals in life.

For example, in order to get into medical school and become a physician, you have to complete four years of undergraduate pre-med university studies, then assuming you have the grades to apply, undergo a rigorous screening and interview process to get into a four-year medical school program. This is usually followed by anywhere from three to six years of residency training, depending on which specialty you wish to practice. All in all, that is potentially fourteen years of education after high school that are required to becoming a practicing physician. This does not include the years of education you receive by treating patients in your practice. For many students, this sacrifice of time and effort is worth it for the privilege of becoming a practicing physician.

In order to climb Mount Everest, you must undergo years of endurance and strength training in addition to learning the technical climbing skills required to reach the summit of the world's highest peak. This does not include the mental toughness, relentless courage, and emotional intelligence required to undertake such an endeavor. However, for many mountaineers and adventurers, making this effort is worth the privilege of being able to say that you summited Mount Everest.

Similarly, the healing journey has its own challenges and obstacles along the way which must be faced if you are to reap the rewards of this journey at the deepest level.

KEY POINTS

1. The healing journey is often a daunting and arduous road that forces you to face your deepest fears and many challenges; however, if it is engaged with unswerving conviction, the rewards are immeasurable and where it takes you is indescribable.
2. The healing journey is an exploration into the inner realms of your being, as it is without destination as it is infinite, and reveals more of its brilliance as you plunge further into its depths.

Chapter 25

The Common Thread Through the Healing Process

Healing is not an easy journey to be on. It takes dedication, perseverance, and an unrelenting desire for nothing short of becoming whole again.

I have laid out the path in this book, but by no means is it a straight path. It is bound to have twists, turns, and detours along the way, as well as potholes and other obstacles. Competing interests will seek your attention and try to deter you.

No two people will have the same exact journey, as it will be shaped by each individual's experiences, personal history, relationships, and the mental and emotional baggage that each of us carry in our own lives.

It is for this reason that each person's healing journey is a unique expression of their being, much like a symphony or a painting is a musician's or an artist's unique expression of their creativity. No matter where your healing journey takes you, both within yourself and in the outer world, one common thread links every step of the unveiling process: love.

The healing journey is ultimately about love. Love is the essence of who you are, the source from which you arose, and the destination to which you will return. Your intention to heal arises out of love. Love is the basis of your life's mission. It fuels your intention, since it is for the greater good of the whole. Love also forms the basis of your connection to yourself, others, nature, the earth, and the entire universe.

All your limiting beliefs can be traced back to a lack of self-love, for when you love yourself beyond measure, you do not perceive any limits to who you are and what is possible. Your emotional blocks arise from not fully experiencing the full spectrum of emotions that life throws at you through different situations.

What you will find is when you feel your emotions fully, you are able to love yourself fully and completely. Any story that you have contrived around your life experiences, and with which you identify, obscures your true essence of light and love. Once you unravel those stories, you allow the light and love within to shine forth.

One of the key ways to raise your vibration is through active self-love and loving others unconditionally. Being the love that you are keeps you in the flow. Love is the essence of the void you dance with when you embrace the unknown. When you unveil your true nature, you create your life and your health from a place of pure love. The healing journey begins and ends with love.

KEY POINTS

- Love is the common thread throughout the entire healing process.

CHAPTER 26

WHERE TO BEGIN THE JOURNEY OF HEALING

To reach the first step in the healing process, intention, you must come from a place of self-love. If you do not love yourself, healing will be challenging for you.

I find that many patients suffering with a chronic disease lack self-love, and it can be difficult to change that paradigm after becoming used to living that way. Paradoxically, once you eliminate your limiting beliefs, remove your emotional blocks, and unravel the stories you identify with, you clear a path for the love that you are to shine forth. It becomes easier to raise your vibration, get into the flow, and embrace the unknown, which are the latter stages in the healing journey. But you need some degree of self-love to even get to the point of setting the intention to heal.

So how do you resolve this healing paradox? You resolve it through awareness. Awareness is the key to getting someone to a place where they can start to heal by setting their intention.

Let's discuss this in some detail.

What is awareness? Awareness is the key tool through which we navigate our life situations. Awareness is a type of knowing, but it is deeper than simply knowing as it also involves focused attention. This focused attention can be directed toward anything within ourselves or outside ourselves.

Unfortunately, most people's attention is directed toward things that do not matter, such as what others think of them, their failures from the past, their worries about the future and what could possibly go wrong, and other aspects of negative thinking. Indeed, the goal of awareness is not to try to change your thoughts and emotions and how you interact with the world; it is to illuminate what lies within in order to impact what lies without.

The process of illuminating your inner world through focused attention will help bring everything to the surface, including your doubts, your fears, your regrets, your perceived failures, where you are not living with integrity with your values, and where you fall short of your own expectations of where you should be in different areas of your life.

The first step to changing anything in your personal paradigm is to engage the focused attention we call awareness. Therefore, if you are not yet at the stage of setting your intention and establishing your powerful why, start simply with awareness.

The simple practice of awareness can give you glimpses of who you truly are and start you on the healing journey. In fact, all healing is simply becoming aware of who you truly are in your core essence and stripping away the layers of who you are not. This is what we have been doing throughout this book through the process I have been describing.

The process of becoming aware simply starts with giving focused attention to your thoughts and emotions without judging them and expecting them to be different than what they are. Let your thoughts and emotions flow effortlessly into the field of your awareness, like a soft, murmuring brook on a quiet summer's day. You may recognize this process as being similar to the process of inner flow from the chapter on flow, but in this context, an awareness practice is meant to illuminate the truth of all that you hold within you.

You may discover negative thoughts, the source of limiting beliefs. You may discover trapped emotions and emotional blocks that have yet to be removed and that's okay. The key to healing is becoming aware of how these entities lodge in your body and create symptoms that eventually lead to disease. You cannot heal until you find the source of what ails you. This is what awareness is all about.

Once you have illuminated your inner world through awareness you may then wish to embark on the healing journey by starting with intention.

Even if you find that you are not yet ready for this first stage, it is okay. It may be a sign that your illness is serving some greater purpose, and it may not be the right time for you to transcend it. In the end, nobody can take your healing journey for you, and you have to be ready to take this journey before you embark on it.

Each step of the healing process requires awareness through intense focus. This is difficult for most people, because whatever we want to accomplish in our lives, there are also many distractions vying for our attention, including television, the internet, social media, and chasing after material things. This is the challenge of healing, but that can be said of anything we want to accomplish in life that is worth the effort. To achieve anything worthwhile in life requires intense focus.

So start off by illuminating your thoughts and emotions and becoming aware of where your attention lies in the moment. You can then direct it to what truly matters, which in this case means the next step you must take in the healing process.

You focus on what you want to achieve by eliminating your mental clutter. Journaling is a good way to accomplish this, as discussed in an earlier chapter. It allows you to get your thoughts down on paper so they do not occupy your mind's attention, allowing you to focus on what is most important to you in the moment. Practice journaling daily. The end of the day is usually a good time to do it, as it allows you to clear your mental clutter so you are free of distractions and can start the next day with clarity of focus.

There is no proper way to journal. All you have to have is a notebook or inexpensive exercise book, a pen or a laptop, at least ten minutes of undistracted time, and the willingness to document all of the thoughts and emotions that have permeated your consciousness throughout the day. This can be an incredibly liberating and enlightening experience, and I encourage everyone to do it, even if they are not engaged in the healing process.

KEY POINTS

1. The healing process always starts with awareness, which is a focused attention on your inner world and what lies within that realm.
2. Each step of the healing process requires deep awareness through intense focus.
3. Journaling is an excellent way of clearing mental clutter and cultivating clarity of focus and can be an incredibly liberating daily practice.

CHAPTER 27

The Pathless Path

I have been talking about how the journey of healing is without destination and is an ongoing journey. However, it goes beyond this. The journey of healing is not a linear path; it is actually nonlinear in nature.

Healing may seem like a linear path because of the way I have described it in this book. However, the only reason it appears linear is because language is a limited means of describing anything in life and does not do justice to the true essence of the entity being discussed.

The truth is that there is no specific sequence of steps on the healing path. The entire process could happen in an instant and completely collapse your perception of reality, or the process could take years or an entire lifetime. Time is relative and not an absolute reality, so the perceived time on the path is irrelevant.

All that matters is that, when you are ready and willing, you take steps along the path and realize that the path to your healing is not necessarily a direct path.

This path will challenge you more than anything you have experienced in your lifetime, which is why few people ever dare to tread this path. The path is initially difficult because of all of the prior conditioning and baggage you have to burn through. But once you push through the initial resistance and struggle, you eventually find that it becomes part of your natural flow state and you travel the path effortlessly.

You may still face twists and turns and many other obstacles along the way, but you will be able to navigate these with ease after you reach an initial threshold on the path. Your threshold will be determined by where in your life you are stuck, whether it is with setting your intention and finding your powerful why, your limiting beliefs, your emotional blocks, or identifying with the stories in your life situation. Most of us will have some degree of all of these thresholds to cross on the healing path.

As I mentioned earlier in this book, the healing journey continues to spiral onto itself and early steps that you took may often need to be revisited and reengaged multiple times. The beauty is that each time you engage in any of the steps on the healing journey, you go deeper than you did previously and gain more insight and self-knowledge with each pass. This reveals more of your true nature and allows more of your self-illusion to drop away. You come closer to wholeness as you engage the process more fully and deeply, which is the essence of healing.

The goal of the healing journey is to reveal to you that you were never ill or broken to begin with and that being healed is your natural state. It is only the illusions and falsehood that you have accumulated through your life's journey that lead you away from your true nature and reinforce the paradigm of chronic disease that a lot of people suffer with.

The beauty of life's journey is that it is always trying to lead you back to your true nature, and your illness is just a signpost to show you that you have deviated away from who you truly are. There are no mistakes, no problems, and nothing to regret in life. Everything that you experience and suffer through in this world is just there to show you the way back to your true self, your whole self, your naturally healed self.

KEY POINTS

- The healing journey is a nonlinear process that takes you deeper into your true nature and closer to wholeness the more you engage the process.

CHAPTER 28

WHY SOME PATIENTS JUST CANNOT HEAL

When I tell my patients and clients that there is a way they can be healed, they often look at me dumbfounded and think that I am crazy. They ask, after living with their disease for many years, how can they possibly transcend it fully and completely?

Even when I tell them that I'm not talking about cure but about experiencing their illness in the context of rediscovering their wholeness, they are still skeptical. The problem is that they are seeing their situation from a very limited viewpoint: past experience.

Most of my patients have not considered that they are "multidimensional beings"; indeed, they do not even know what this means. They do not consider their thoughts, emotions, and spirit as aspects of their being or their experience on this earth in a physical body. Their bodies, their medical conditions, and their symptoms are the limits of their experiential reality.

You can imagine how far a stretch it is for most of my patients and clients to go beyond their limited conception of reality and see themselves as infinite beings who can achieve incredible feats in this earthly life. This is through no fault of their own; it results from their upbringing and life experiences, where all they may have seen is lack, limitation, and limited potential.

But if I can get my patients to do some of the exercises described in this book and access their inner realms, I am able to turn their limited conception of reality upside down and reframe it in the context of their true nature and their whole being. At that point, they start to see their potential and the infinite possibilities available to them, including optimal health and living disease-free.

I have stated that healing is not about cure; it is about realigning all levels of your being to create the best circumstances for your condition to be effectively treated, with a potential decrease and elimination of all your symptoms. I do not take this claim lightly, but I do know that it is not only possible but the most probable outcome if you follow the journey outlined in this book.

For most people, what is required is a suspension of belief, a leap of faith into the unknown of pure possibility. If you think about it, you have nothing to lose by taking this leap of faith, except for potential disappointment if what I have been telling you is not true.

But even if you do not believe anything you have read in this book, is it still not worth it to take this leap and risk disappointment? Is it not better than living with the burden of chronic disease and all of its symptoms, manifestations, and the burden of pharmaceutical treatment?

As I intimated earlier, if at this point you still want to hold onto your illness and are not willing to consider the possibility of being healed, it is because the illness is likely serving some purpose in your life.

But what greater purpose could being sick serve?

For some people, illness may be a way of keeping their mind distracted from other problems in their lives. For other people, illness may be a way to alleviate loneliness, as they get to visit their family doctor, specialists, and occasionally get admitted to the hospital, where they also interact with nurses as well as other hospital staff. Illness may give some people a sense of purpose, as it is something they need to conquer. The problem is that if they ever do eventually overcome their condition, they will lose their sense of purpose. For some people, illness may be a means of getting attention from spouses, children, extended family, and friends.

These are just a few of the many reasons why someone may want to remain ill. This is why I have said that everyone can be led to the path that begins the healing journey, but each person has to make the decision to embark on this journey on their own.

What I have found is that most people who are able to discover and cultivate their life's mission as an expression of their higher purpose will want to embark on the healing journey. This is why finding your life's mission is a key part of setting the intention to heal.

KEY POINTS

1. There are many reasons why someone may not want to engage in the healing process.
2. In these cases the illness is usually serving some purpose in the individual's life situation.
3. An integral part of getting someone to engage the healing process is to help them discover and cultivate their life's mission as an expression of a higher purpose, which is a crucial aspect of setting the intention to heal.

CHAPTER 29

THIS IS NOT ABOUT YOU

Healing is not just about you. It is about healing the whole of humanity, which is currently suffering in unprecedented ways.

The burden of humanity's suffering includes the growing gap between the world's richest and poorest people, which leads to severe economic disparity around the globe and poverty. This in turn leads to global regional conflict, war and terrorism, increasing disconnection and violence amongst our youth, and the growing illusion of separation amongst the world's population, despite being more connected through advancing technology. Humanity is also inflicting suffering on the earth in the form of climate change and destruction of the planet's various delicate ecosystems in the name of corporate greed for profit.

Why is humanity experiencing such incredible suffering?

The reason is that each and every one of us who make up the body of humanity is living through some degree of unresolved personal pain and grief.

This pain arises from many causes. These include childhood physical and emotional abuse; not being fully and unconditionally loved while growing up; being brainwashed into false beliefs by our flawed educational systems; addictions resulting from the inability or unwillingness to go deep within; falsely believing that the source of our wealth and abundance lies outside ourselves, which leads to financial struggle; strained and challenging relationships with others who are broken and in pain; living with chronic disease and physical pain, with no clear means of healing; and seeing ourselves as limited beings with limited potential.

The reason we are all suffering is because we have not been given the tools to heal ourselves from the issues mentioned above. This is what this book is about, but its application goes well beyond healing chronic disease, as these principles can be applied to healing any area of your life so that you can flourish from a deep internal place of wellness.

The problem is that it is not enough for each of us to heal in isolation; this healing has to spread globally, to every individual in the collective body of humanity, if we are to right the wrongs and heal the ills that humanity suffers from. The reason why humanity continues to suffer is because our world leaders, many of whom are suffering themselves, are trying to solve our global problems through external means, whether it be war, terrorism, economic disparity, poverty, slavery in the form of human trafficking, or climate change.

Just as we cannot heal from chronic diseases through medications and surgery, without a multidimensional, multifaceted approach to healing, the world's problems will never be solved through solely external solutions, as they do not address an individual's daily inner crises. The well-known famous physicist Einstein was quoted as saying that you cannot solve a problem with the same level of consciousness that created it.

All the pain, angst, and turmoil that we carry inside becomes externalized and manifests as the global crises that we face in this day and age. What we see in the world is a reflection of the collective inner state of all of humanity, which speaks volumes to the degree of anguish and torment we are all experiencing. This is not any one person's fault, because very few of us have been taught how to live in alignment with our true nature.

Few people realize that their inner state reflects the outer state they experience in the world, and yet so many of us want desperately for humanity to change. It is important, therefore, that the healing process be taught not only as a means to self-healing but also as a means to effect change in one's environment.

Evidence that our collective inner state affects the external environment is supported by the Washington Peace Study, which took place from June 7 to July 30, 1993.[1] Even though this is an older study, its results are still relevant today. For this study, a 27-member project review board was set up comprising independent scientists and leading citizens. Their task was to ensure objectivity and research rigor by reviewing and approving the research protocol and then subsequently monitoring the research process.

Washington's immediate history at this time showed that during the first five months of the year prior to the research project, violent crime had been steadily increasing. This increase continued on into the first two weeks of the project, when homicides actually continued to increase.

The intervention involved having a number of practitioners of transcendental meditation (TM) engage in meditation practice daily during the study period. The numbers of these practitioners started out at 800 and grew to 4,000 by the end of the study period.

The results showed a 23.3 percent drop in violent crime over the study period, with the statistical probability of less than 2 in 1 billion that this result could reflect chance variation in crime levels. In addition, the researchers tested their findings for other possible causes of crime reduction, such as temperature, precipitation, weekends, and police and community anti-crime activities and found that the drop in crime could not be attributed to any of these other possibilities.

In fact, forty-nine research projects conducted in numerous countries around the world over the last forty years show that regular group meditation reduced war deaths, reduced terrorism, reduced crime rates, resulted in less emergency calls, fewer suicides and accidents, less alcohol consumption—concrete proof that our collective inner state affects our external environment.

These studies only looked at meditation, a means of achieving inner flow that is one of the steps in the healing process outlined in this book. Imagine if a threshold of individuals were to engage in the entire healing process, from intention to creation. This would surely have an exponentially greater effect than meditation alone on crime, war, terrorism, and environmental decimation.

The sad thing is that the majority of humanity is caught up in the false premise that we can solve our global problems through the traditional means that we have been trying to employ for years. But if we look at the world we live in today, it is painfully obvious that this is not true. We just keep spinning our wheels trying hopelessly to achieve results that can only be obtained by going deep within, as outlined in this book. This is why it is crucial, not just for our own individual healing but for the healing of humanity's ills, that the process outlined in this book be widely disseminated to as many people as possible. I have already outlined in an earlier chapter how this can be done; however, I would like to take this farther here.

I have outlined how to get people interested in engaging in their own individual healing process at grassroots level. Now I would like to get deeply personal and delve deeper into the issues that surround our global problems.

The sad fact is that there are people who actually benefit from the state of affairs as they are. For example, war and terrorism support the military and defense industries, which feed the profits of corporations involved in manufacturing the weapons and arms needed to wage war and fight terrorism. It is not far fetched to surmise that somehow, even if indirectly, these corporations promote, for their own selfish profit, the political turmoil and international tensions that create the circumstances resulting in war and terrorism. Political leaders may also stand to benefit from conflict, by oppressing the majority in order to protect the financial interests of the minority.

The political leaders and CEOs of these corporations are shortsighted and blinded by their limiting beliefs, subconscious and emotional blocks, identification with their life stories, low vibrational frequency, and feeling disconnected from others and nature. As a result, they are not in the flow, and their fear of the unknown leads them to seek personal financial security at the expense of others.

The way to engage these individuals in the healing process and change their perspective is to seek them out and show them how this process could benefit them or someone close to them. This is not hard to do since everyone either suffers from or knows someone who suffers from a chronic disease, chronic anxiety, or the effects of stress. You have to be anxious and stressed to want to inflict pain on others for your own personal gain.

Once the people in power start to realize how the healing process can help them, they will naturally want to move away from and eventually stop the activities they engage in that perpetuate other people's suffering. The key is to get this information into their hands so it can become the focus of their attention. This can be done by learning the information in this book and then engaging others in this process, especially those who are politically and economically influential.

There are many means to do this, including sending the key players emails, petitions, and engaging mainstream and alternative media and social media. There will be resistance to something new and innovative at first, but with relentless persistence, this information will eventually disseminate to corporations, government offices, nonprofit organizations, educational institutions, and community associations.

Even if this information is initially ignored by those who have power and control, it will take hold at grassroots levels in these organizations and slowly filter its way up through the hierarchical structure. A process that is beneficial for all, no matter what their physical, mental, emotional, or spiritual situation is, can only be ignored for so long before it garners the attention of leaders in all realms of society.

Once the benefits of this healing process start to be realized, they will naturally attract attention and reach those who need it the most, including, hopefully, influential leaders. Eventually, those leaders with influence over others in society will change their choices and decisions in a way that is beneficial for the greater good of humanity and beneficial for our planet.

There is another, even more powerful way that our inner state can affect our external reality. In the chapter on intention, I have already discussed how we are all connected. This connection permeates to the deepest levels of who we are, and any change in our own inner state will naturally realign those of others in our immediate environment. They, in turn, will effect similar changes in other people in their surroundings in a healing chain reaction.

In this way, the healing process, once initiated in a handful of individuals, can exponentially spread to others, influencing those at the highest levels of society, once it reaches a tipping point. In this way, the whole of humanity can be healed once a threshold of individuals has experienced the healing process. This is my ultimate hope and dream for this healing process, and I feel that it is inevitable once it takes hold in society.

KEY POINTS

1. The collective inner state of the individuals who make up the whole of humanity reflects the external circumstances that we see in the world today.
2. The healing process is, ultimately, for the benefit of humanity as a whole and the planet, which is suffering at the hands of broken, misidentified, and suffering individuals who compromise the bulk of humanity.
3. Because meditation has been proven to have a positive effect on the immediate environment, the healing process, once engaged in by a threshold of individuals, is sure to have a greater exponential positive effect on the immediate community, greater society and, ultimately, the planet as a whole.

CHAPTER 30

Touching the Infinite and Achieving the Impossible

The final stage in the healing journey is embracing the unknown. When this is done fully and completely, without fear or hesitation, you realize yourself as the infinite being that you truly are. You see yourself as no longer separate from the infinite universe and a creator of your own physical reality. It is in this final phase that you realize your true unlimited potential to heal from anything you may be suffering from. This is where the impossible morphs into the realm of possibility and the impossible loses its meaning.

Some may call this stage self-actualization, awakening, satori, or enlightenment. You can call it what you want but, in actuality, this is just the next stage in our evolution as human beings on planet Earth.

We needed to forget in order to remember. We needed to be lost in order to be found. We needed to take the form of dense physical bodies in order to realize the higher levels of our being, which are not separate from the universe, the Higher Power or God if you prefer. This is the stage of full mastery of life, when you realize that your illness was given to you as a gift to either gently nudge you or violently thrust you into this timeless awareness. This is where you realize your eternal nature and that what once appeared to be impossible was simply just outside the realm of your understanding of the nature of reality.

Most people only reach this type of profound realization after death; however, it is possible to reach it while you are still alive through the process I have outlined in this book. You now have all the tools you need to heal from anything that ails you and anything you may be suffering from. It is up to you to do something with this knowledge and, if you're not yet ready to help yourself, pass this wisdom onto someone who you think could benefit from it.

Not a day goes by that I don't encounter several people whom I know would benefit from what I have shared in this book. And so begins the greater journey of healing everyone on the planet and healing the planet itself, which is only suffering at the hands of broken and misidentified human beings.

So, go forth and spread this wisdom wide and far—if not for your own benefit, then for the benefit of someone you care about and, ultimately, for the benefit of the earth itself.

Acknowledgments

I would like to acknowledge the many authors and speakers who have been influential and inspirational in my journey to write this book. These include, in no particular order: Eckhart Tolle, Bernie Siegel, Neale Donald Walsch, Deepak Chopra, Mark Nepo, Michael Bernard Beckwith, Gangaji, Matt Kahn, Gay Henricks, Bruce Lipton, Gregg Braden, Guy Finley, Wayne Dyer, Carolyn Myss, Louise Hay, Anita Moorjani, Gabor Maté, Kelly Turner, John Robbins, and Joel Fuhrman.

I would like to thank my mentors in deep nature connection who introduced me to a whole new world of inner and outer awareness. They are Skeet Sutherland of Sticks and Stones Wilderness School in Ontario, Canada and Chris Gilmour, both of whom mentored me in wilderness survival and primitive living skills, and Alexis Burnett of Earth Tracks in Ontario, Canada who mentored me in the ancient art of tracking.

I would like to thank one of my mentors in my life's journey, Rose Saroyan, who proofread my book before it got to the publisher.

I would like to thank Sabine Weeke, the acquisitions editor, and Findhorn Press who saw the value and importance of my work and have provided me the means to get it out to the world. I would like to thank Nicky Leach, the copy editor at Findhorn Press, for her superb editing of the book you now hold.

I would like to thank my mother and father who instilled in me the value of hard work and relentless persistence in achieving any goal that I set my mind to.

I would like to thank my wonderful wife, Reema Niaz, without whose patience during the writing process this book would not have been possible.

I dedicate this book to my three beautiful children: Sofie, Aariz, and Alina.

Notes

Chapter 2

1. Centers for Disease Control and Prevention. "Chronic Disease Overview: Costs of Chronic Disease." Centers for Disease Control and Prevention website. Available at *http://www.cdc.gov/nccdphp/overview.htm*

2. Mensah G, Brown D. "An overview of cardiovascular disease burden in the United States." Health Aff 2007; 26:38-48.

3. American Diabetes Association. "Direct and Indirect Costs of Diabetes in the United States." American Diabetes Association website. Available at *http://www.diabetes.org/diabetes-statistics/*

4. National Heart, Lung, and Blood Institute. "Morbidity and Mortality: 2004 Chart Book on Cardiovascular, Lung, and Blood Diseases." Bethesda, MD: National Institutes of Health, 2004.

5. Alzheimer's Association. "Alzheimer's Disease Facts and Figures 2007." Alzheimer's Association website. Available at *http://www.alz.org/national/ documents/Report_2007 FactsandFigures.pdf*

Chapter 23

1. *www.cancer.ca*

Chapter 29

1. Hagelin JS; Orme-Johnson DW; Rainforth M; Cavanaugh KL; Alexander CN; Shatkin SF; Davies JL; Hughs AO; Ross E; "Effects of Group Practice of the Transcendental Meditation Program on Preventing Violent Crime in Washington, D.C.: Results of the National Demonstration Project, June–July 1993," D.C.Institute of Science, Technology and Public Policy Technical Report 94:1, 1994. Social Indicators Research 1999; vol. 47 issue 2: 153-201.

Resources

Alexander, Eben. *Proof of Heaven: A Neurosurgeon's Journey into the Afterlife.* Simon and Schuster, 2013.

Braden, Gregg. *Deep Truth: Igniting the Memory of Our Origin, History, Destiny, and Fate.* Hay House, 2012.

____ *The Divine Matrix: Bridging Time, Space, Miracles, and Belief.* Hay House, 2008.

____ *The Spontaneous Healing of Belief: Shattering the Paradigm of False Limits.* Hay House, 2009.

____ *Resilience from the Heart: The Power to Thrive in Life's Extremes.* Hay House, 2015.

Chopra, Deepak. *Perfect Health.* Harmony, 2001.

____ *Quantum Healing.* Bantam, 2015.

____ *The Seven Spiritual Laws Of Success.* Amber-Allen Publishing, 2010.

Chopra, Deepak, Tanzi, Rudolph E. *Super Genes: Unlock the Astonishing Power of Your DNA for Optimum Health and Well-Being.* Harmony, 2015.

Dyer, Wayne. *Excuses Begone! How to Change Lifelong, Self-Defeating Thinking Habits.* Hay House, 2011.

____ *Inspiration: Your Ultimate Calling.* Hay House, 2007.

____ *The Power of Intention.* Hay House, 2005.

____ *There's a Spiritual Solution to Every Problem.* Quill, 2003.

____ *Wisdom of the Ages: 60 Days to Enlightenment.* William Morrow Paperbacks, 2002.

____ *You'll See It When You Believe It: The Way to Your Personal Transformation.* William Morrow Paperbacks, 2001.

Finley, Guy. *The Essential Laws of Fearless Living: Find the Power to Never Feel Powerless Again.* Red Wheel/Weiser, 2008.

____ *The Secret of Letting Go.* Llewellyn Publications, 2007.

Fuhrman, Joel. *The End of Diabetes: The Eat to Live Plan to Prevent and Reverse Diabetes*. HarperOne, 2014.

___ *The End of Heart Disease: The Eat to Live Plan to Prevent and Reverse Heart Disease*. HarperOne, 2016.

___ *Super Immunity: The Essential Nutrition Guide for Boosting Your Body's Defenses to Live Longer, Stronger, and Disease Free*. HarperOne, 2013.

Gangaji. *The Diamond in Your Pocket: Discovering Your True Radiance*. Sounds True, 2007.

___ *Hidden Treasure: Uncovering the Truth in Your Life Story*. TarcherPerigee, 2012.

Hay, Louise. *Heal Your Body*. Hay House, 1984.

___ *You Can Heal Your Life*. Hay House, 1984.

Hendricks, Gay. *The Big Leap: Conquer Your Hidden Fear and Take Life to the Next Level*. HaperOne, 2010.

___ *Conscious Breathing: Breathwork for Health, Stress Release, and Personal Mastery*. Bantam, 1995.

Kahn, Matt. *Whatever Arises, Love That: A Love Revolution That Begins with You*. Sounds True, 2016.

Lipton, Bruce. *The Biology of Belief: Unleashing the Power of Consciousness, Matter & Miracles*. Hay House, 2016.

Mate, Gabor. *In the Realm of Hungry Ghosts: Close Encounters with Addiction*. North Atlantic Books, 2010.

___ *When the Body Says No: Understanding the Stress-Disease Connection*. Wiley, 2011.

Moorjani, Anita. *Dying To Be Me: My Journey from Cancer, to Near Death, to True Healing*. Hay House, 2014.

Myss, Carolyn. *Anatomy of the Spirit: The Seven Stages of Power and Healing*. Harmony, 1996.

___ *The Creation of Health: The Emotional, Psychological, and Spiritual Responses That Promote Health and Healing*. Harmony, 1998.

___ *Why People Don't Heal and How They Can*. Harmony, 1998.

Neill, Michael. *The Inside-Out Revolution: The Only Thing You Need to Know to Change Your Life Forever*. Hay House, 2013.

___ *The Space Within: Finding Your Way Back Home*. Hay House UK, 2016.

Nepo, Mark. *As Far As the Heart Can See: Stories to Illuminate the Soul*. HCI, 2011.

Nepo, Mark. *The Book of Awakening: Having the Life You Want by Being Present to the Life You Have.* Conari Press, 2000.

___ *The Endless Practice: Becoming Who You Were Born to Be.* Atria Books, 2014.

___ *The Exquisite Risk: Daring to Live an Authentic Life.* Harmony, 2006.

___ *Finding Inner Courage.* Conari Press, 2011.

___ *Inside the Miracle: Enduring Suffering, Approaching Wholeness.* Sounds True, 2015.

Robbins, John. *Diet for a New America.* HJ Kramer, 1998.

___ *Healthy at 100: The Scientifically Proven Secrets of the World's Healthiest and Longest-Lived Peoples.* Ballantine Books, 2007.

___ *The Food Revolution: How Your Diet Can Help Save Your Life and Our World.* Conari Press, 2010.

Siegel, Bernie S. *How to Live Between Office Visits: A Guide to Life, Love and Health.* HarperCollins, 1993.

___ *Love, Medicine and Miracles: Lessons Learned about Self-Healing from a Surgeon's Experience with Exceptional Patients.* HarperPerennial, 1998.

___ *The Art of Healing: Uncovering Your Inner Wisdom and Potential for Self-Healing.* New World Library, 2013.

Tolle, Eckhart. *A New Earth: Awakening to Your Life's Purpose.* Penguin, 2008.

___ *The Power of Now: A Guide to Spiritual Enlightenment.* Namaste Publishing, 2004.

___ *Stillness Speaks.* New World Library, 2003.

Turner, Kelly. *Radical Remission: Surviving Cancer Against All Odds.* HarperOne, 2015.

Walsch, Neale Donald. *Conversations with God: Book 1: An Uncommon Dialogue.* Hodder Paperback, 1997.

___ *Conversations With God: Book 2: An Uncommon Dialogue.* Hampton Roads Publishing Company, 1997.

___ *Conversations With God: Book 3: An Uncommon Dialogue.* Hampton Roads Publishing Company, 1998.

___ *Friendship with God: An Uncommon Dialogue.* TarcherPerigee, 2002.

___ *Home with God: In a Life That Never Ends.* Atria Books, 2007.

___ *When Everything Changes, Change Everything: In a Time of Turmoil, A Pathway to Peace.* Emnin Books, 2011.

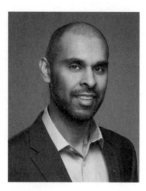

ABOUT THE AUTHOR

Dr. Naeem is a physician specializing in pulmonary and critical care medicine whose intellectual journey has taken him far beyond the confines of conventional medicine. He has practiced in both the United States and Canada over the course of eighteen years, including his training, at the time of this book's publication and has treated tens of thousands of patients.

Over the course of his career, he has realized that the majority of patients with chronic disease do not heal, a percentage of which have no desire to heal. This realization compelled him to dive deeper into the psychology of healing human consciousness, metaphysics, and healing traditions from the past through his own personal research and study to uncover how he can facilitate healing in his patients and clients.

What resulted from this journey is the subject of this book. Dr. Naeem lives with his wife and three children in Mississauga, Ontario, Canada, where he carries on his conventional medical practice, along with teaching, coaching, and consulting on what he has learned.

He can be reached at *wholehealthexpert@gmail.com*. Please visit his website at *naumannaeem.com* for more information on his coaching, consulting, and speaking services.